Love from
Pat

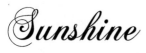

Sunshine

and

Shadow

My Battle with Bipolar Disorder

Mahala Busselle Bishop

iUniverse, Inc.
New York   Bloomington

Sunshine and Shadow
My Battle with Bipolar Disorder

The information, ideas, and suggestions in this book are not intended as a substitute for professional medical advice. Before following any suggestions contained in this book, you should consult your personal physician. Neither the author nor the publisher shall be liable or responsible for any loss or damage allegedly arising as a consequence of your use or application of any information or suggestions in this book.

iUniverse books may be ordered through booksellers or by contacting:

iUniverse
1663 Liberty Drive
Bloomington, IN 47403
www.iuniverse.com
1-800-Authors (1-800-288-4677)

Because of the dynamic nature of the Internet, any Web addresses or links contained in this book may have changed since publication and may no longer be valid. The views expressed in this work are solely those of the author and do not necessarily reflect the views of the publisher, and the publisher hereby disclaims any responsibility for them.

ISBN: 978-1-4401-3740-2 (sc)
ISBN: 978-1-4401-3741-9 (e-book)

Printed in the United States of America

iUniverse rev. date: 4/06/2009

Dedication

To Harriet, John, Mandy and Scott for their unceasing support and to Don, for sticking with me through terrible times and writing these wonderful poems.

Contents

Introduction

I am a manic depressive and suffer from bipolar disorder -- the two names for this awful disease are interchangeable. As I move through the years of my tunnel of horror, my goal is to help people better understand the nature of this debilitating and incurable disease. It is my hope and belief that I am uniquely qualified to describe the inside of both facets of the illness – mania and depression -- to fully inform readers without overwhelming them with medical jargon. As the disease came on in my fifties (very unusual), I had already had much more life experience than most victims, I have a love affair with writing, a wonderful education, and multitudes of notes from several manic episodes.

I am not unique in having vast residues of guilt, shame and violation due to my obscenely hurtful actions while manic. But the world needs to know that our guilt is misplaced, that we are not monsters. We could just as well have cancer or diabetes. Being a victim of manic depression is not our fault.   Public fear of and anger towards us can be explained by ignorance, and alleviated by information and understanding.

There is so much stigma attached to mental illness in general, manic depression in particular, and there are many reasons for it, one of which is that it is apparently unbelievably frightening to be around someone with acute mania. As a victim, I cannot begin to imagine I could be terrifying, that my (to me) incredibly lucid speech appears completely crazy to everyone in earshot, that even emails give it all away. One's self-perception has disappeared.

Everyone is affected by a person in the throes of a manic episode: observers, friends, especially family. My goal in writing this book is that a wide spectrum of people will read what I have written, learn about this illness, realize that it ultimately removes all judgment from the brain of its victims. Perhaps with this further information they will think about me and others like me with more compassion and understanding than the amusement and horror with which they observed my antics. And the stigma will gradually lessen.

Before, during and after hospitalizations in 2000, 2003 and 2005, I took reams of notes, always assuring people that I was going to write a book about mental disorders. In the fall of 2005, I began to do research on manic depression. But my commitment to write about my own personal experience became all-important during a workshop serendipitously centered on mental health that I attended with my niece in March of 2006.

In addition to many, many months of research, mostly non-fiction, medical, academic (and therefore often dry and unreadable!), some fictional accounts, I also conducted interviews with friends and family who had been affected closely or from afar by my mania, less so by my depression. (When one is depressed, there is very little social interaction. It's too difficult and requires too much effort.) Some of them agreed to write about our encounters and I have quoted much of their writing.

In conclusion, my goal is to present information that may be new, that in being self-revelatory it gives a graphic description of what being on the inside of a manic mind is like, what depression does to a person – in other words to inform readers about this awful disease in a way they perhaps have not felt nor understood before.

A Quick Tour of Possible Causes of Manic Depression

There are innumerable studies as to the causes of manic depression. It is generally believed that even if genes are not definitely a cause, they pose a risk, acting as "predisposing agents." Having a manic depressive in the family, as I do, is not conclusive, but as David Miklowitz writes, *"it provides one piece of the diagnostic puzzle."*

Many researchers feel that nothing can trigger the disease without the gene or genes: that a genetic tendency towards temperamental instability causes a person's vulnerability to the illness. Some have concluded that the risk to a first-degree relative is up to ten times that of someone without the history.

A person may be born with biological disturbances, vulnerabilities, which though perhaps only dormant, make him susceptible to manic and depressive episodes. Over-and under-production of neurotransmitters and/or abnormality in the nerve cell receptors may be caused by these vulnerabilities.

It seems that one's reactions to stress are affected by these biological disturbances and then the latter create the stress. It was first noted over a century ago that precipitating events (for instance loss, death, crisis) often bring on the beginning of the first episodes, but as time goes on, the vulnerability increases and the actual stress is no longer necessary. The brain that has gone into mania or depression will continue to return to them again and again. I find this tremendously disturbing, as even taking pains to avoid stress will not help stave off other episodes of either side of the disease.

No one seems to know for sure what the causes are, why certain treatments are effective for some and not for others, nor is it understood why an individual is affected by circumstances that leave another untouched. However, few doctors and researchers dispute the fact that manic depression is due to a chemical imbalance and the majority agree that only proper medication will constitute a cure or cause a remission. The good news is that so many are trying to answer these questions.

A Somewhat Brief Biography

I had a heavenly childhood – two loving parents, my father an architect who set off daily from Princeton on the "dinky" to work in New York, my mother the assistant head of an excellent private school. Her job ensured that all four of us could attend. I thought I was the luckiest person in the world – two older sisters and a brother who adored me, friends whose parents often took me to New York for shows and dinners, my own family specializing more in taking us to lectures at Princeton University. Life growing up in the '50's was great.

The school, Miss Fine's, had exacting standards of education and fierce attention to its students. I graduated in a class of 21 in 1961 and was accepted at Radcliffe. The years at school were wonderful, with a close cadre of athletic, intellectual friends, later dances and flirtations with Princeton students mixed in with the serious studies. I was especially pleased to be president of my class in the 11th grade, and then re-elected for senior year (though I missed half of it as an exchange student to Finland with American Field Service).

Languages were my forte from the start, especially French, which I continued at Radcliffe but was bowled over there by an intensely bright, dynamic German teacher. My enthusiasm for his language sent me off to the University of Munich for Junior Year, which turned out to be a great, eye-opening experience, resulting in super fluency with the language and a good vision of much of western Europe. A year later, before I had figured out what to do after college, I was called home as my sister Lucy had tried to commit suicide and was hospitalized.

The diagnosis was manic depression., often referred to now as bipolar disorder. In 1965 few people knew anything about this disease and its horrific consequences. Patients were incarcerated, plied with Thorazine and other numbing drugs, given electric shock. Lithium, the first well-recognized successful treatment, was not accepted in this country until the early seventies.

As we all tried to care for her small boys, we went about our lives in helpless agony, especially my parents, trying to make the right decisions for her care but really having no idea whom to believe, what different hospitals might offer, not knowing how to explain this illness to their friends. Mental illness is still often blamed on bad parenting, so they suffered in silence and guilt. Social stigma was indescribable, and it hasn't improved much. I can only imagine their confusion, as their eldest, most brilliant academically and socially achieving child became someone no one understood. Gradually in the spring of 1966 the mania was tamed.

After a dinner party that summer at William Styron's home on Martha's Vineyard, where I'd had a fine conversation on the porch with Robert Kennedy and his dog Freckles, I went laughing home to my parents, "Oh, guess what, Senator Kennedy asked me what I was doing in September and offered me a choice of three jobs!" I chose the one in Washington, began in his Senate office in September and left two months after his death in June of 1968. I always felt very special to him, having been singled out that evening.

I began as a receptionist, juggling out of work constituents with visiting monarchs. The job was actually very hard and endlessly fun. Taking the Senator for rides around Washington on my large, red motorcycle did not endear me to his secretary and I was relegated to writing legislative and press mail in the back room. Despite my slow shorthand and moderate typing skills, I graduated to secretary to the Administrative Assistant, Joe Dolan, and to working with John Nolan in Advance and Scheduling in the campaign. Two extraordinary men. When the Senator was killed, we had 60 days to close the office. We could have done it in 6. Instead, we used the time to cry and mourn and grieve. I've never stopped, I don't think.

For me these were an extraordinary two years. I'd still be there if he were alive and needed my help in promoting his vision of a better world. The enormity of the loss of the Senator seems to be felt more, not less deeply by the world as these dreadful years pass. I am now convinced that I can date my gradual slide into depression and perhaps into manic depression from that day in 1968.

Unable to imagine living in a country where such a thing could happen, I lit out for Spain, where I was employed as assistant/translator in a graduate program. My English, French, German and improving Spanish made me very useful, but the prospect of a friend's motorcycle trip across North Africa was more intriguing. We bought two huge Triumph Bonnevilles in London, crossed the Pyrenees in late February (that was not fun), traveled across the top of the continent through sandstorms, got arrested in Egypt, bounced on and off ferries up through the Middle East and back to Switzerland. 10,000 miles. Often more fun to look back on than to experience.

A stroke of fortune was my acceptance to the campaign staff of Senator George McGovern in 1970. What a heady time of life and idealism and fabulous, bright people! We never thought we'd lose the election so summarily, if at all. Other political and news jobs eventually lost their luster for me as it began to seem quite clear I needed to do something with my hands. My decision was to leave Washington and become a potter.

After several years of learning how to throw pots and after marrying Don Bishop and moving to Cape Cod to care for his elderly mother, I opened the doors of Spindrift Pottery on the Town Cove in Orleans in 1980 and stayed there for almost 20 years. A constant flow of friends, my dogs, customers, swimmers – so much fun.

In the early '90s, following a course in community

mediation, I turned my attention to opportunities in that field: small claims court, trainings, postal service. It is an incredibly powerful, satisfying process. I always leap at the chance to hone my skills, help others listen to each other and hopefully come to a hitherto impossible agreement.

Since closing Spindrift at the end of the '90's, we have gravitated more and more to Maine, where I have a small pottery showroom and Don has become a sculptor, painter and woodworker, always more of an artist than his wife. In addition to a large summer garden, the pottery, our boats, I have turned my attention to teaching English as a foreign language. Having done a course on line at home and then traveled to Argentina for on the spot training, I am now certified to do what I've enjoyed so much doing over the past years. This looks to be the next step in my somewhat varied career.

Chapter One:

A First Glimpse of Mania

I felt great that May of 1994, right before Memorial Day weekend as I rushed to make pots for the fair coming up, to plan for the expected masses arriving on the Cape, and to ready the bed and breakfast wing of the house. By now Spindrift Pottery was an institution in Orleans, the first stop for many summer visitors. My dogs lolled around all day watching me throw pots outdoors. There were endless fascinating conversations with friends and strangers and interestingly enough, distinctive themes developed each summer about retirement or mothers, for instance. The subjects would mysteriously reintroduce themselves over and over, and everyone had something to contribute. Strangers would find themselves at the shop for hours. Friday afternoons Spindrift hosted potluck wine parties, enjoyed by diverse groups.

Days were long – often 9 or 10 hours at the shop itself, where for the most part I would be throwing pots, then hours before and after making glazes, doing the glazing and firing at home in my workspace in the garage. The summer fairs were not only important financially but even more to entice people who had only seen the sign to make their way back to my hidden location.

In addition to the wonderful arguments and discussions that took place at Spindrift Pottery, I learned so much from our bed and breakfast guests – often of different nationalities and usually clinicians or psychologists studying at a near-by symposium. There wasn't much time to visit with them, but the interaction was more important than the much-needed income.

Don had less to do with the guests than I did – he was more concerned with his elderly mother. We had been married in 1978 and moved shortly thereafter to Cape Cod to care for her. Blessed with a sunny personality, loving friends and family Don is a supremely self-confident, artistic and intelligent individual. He had spent his youth on a farm in Vermont, learning to ride wonderfully and then in college to run around a track like a rabbit. After a few false starts after graduation from Amherst, like law school and another one selling mutual funds in Geneva, Don enjoyed a four-year stint as business manager of a new school in Phoenix – the job that led him to his major love, France.

Don lived in France for years, first in the center of the country with his first wife and two small daughters teaching English as a second language, then as Athletic

Director at the American School of Paris. In addition to that job, he taught everything under the sun including French, rock climbing, and photography. When we met, through my sister Harriet, who had also been teaching in Paris, Don was at a private school in New Jersey, teaching French.

When we moved to the Cape in 1979, Don thought he'd try something new and went into real estate. His office was in front of a small building on the cove, and when a painter came in to inquire about renting it, his question to me was, *"Why don't you open a shop with her? What are you doing with your pottery anyway?"* The beginning of the era of Spindrift Pottery!

Why my mood began to speed up that May is such a mystery – I had just turned 50, three decades after the normal onset of mental disorder – but my inordinate cheer, lack of interest in even my favorite foods (with a very obvious weight loss), my incessant chatter alarmed my friends. I sloughed it off to how hard I was working to make pots for the first big weekend of the summer, but my friends didn't buy it.

*"You know, Pol, you were **way** more than 'hypomanic' that May,"* said my long-time close friend Susan after she'd read the first draft of this book. *"Don't you remember that day at the house on Doane Road when you and Dave had a **12** hour conversation? And what about the fashion show you insisted we needed to see when you pulled all your clothes out of the closet and tried them on for our whole family? I wondered why you thought the kids would be interested – I think they were about 7 and 8 at the time. Knowing you*

as well as I do and especially knowing how little you care about clothes and your looks in general, something was way, way off."

The job of taking action and dealing with my increasingly self-destructive behavior fell to my most pro-active friend, Marcia, who recently wrote the following:

"So, when Polly came to my sweet sea side cottage on the beach, I thought she was coming to seek refuge from the world, to be in touch with that strengthening source readily available at the edge of the ocean. When she announced that her clothes were in the car and she was staying the night so she could wake looking at the sea, I continued to think she had come for refreshment of the spirit, but Mykee noticed that she was talking to the food over dinner.

"When in the morning she admitted to no sleep at all, I became concerned. She went off to her business of making pottery and then I began to receive phone calls from our friends asking if I had seen Pol and what did I think and what could be done…she wasn't making sense. And what am I to do, I thought. Well, believe in the stable Polly, and bring her back. I was certain that other, stable friend was around some corner of time. I felt worry, not fear.

"I called her and said something like, 'Pol, you do not seem okay to me or to some of our friends. Who would you trust to help you?' "None of those people who want to put me on drugs or lock me up," she said. "Louisa." *Louisa is a mutual friend, a psychiatric social worker, who rearranged her schedule and came to help. I was relieved and secure in the knowledge that Polly would return to her old self.*

Permanently. And that Louisa would be able to midwife the rebirth. I was wrong. Healing was not to be an absolute."

Blissfully unaware as I was of the numerous concerned conversations between a whole gang of close friends, I was amazed when Louisa appeared at my door, saying she was worried about me and that it was costing her $400 to come tell me that. I laughed and told her, "Louisa, you are being ridiculous. Why don't you just let me lie down and take a nap, I've just been working too hard." But as she was such a good friend, she exacted a promise from me to do whatever she asked – it turned out it was to go to the doctor. Since I try to live up to commitments, even though I knew this was a total waste of time, we went and ended up in the Emergency Room.

During the several frustrating hours in which Louisa had tried to deal with my resistance to seeking medical attention, she remembers, *"You were full of some sort of critical revelation about the universe. You were really hard to keep up with. All the theories that kept pouring out of you were somewhat convincing but crazy. And under no circumstances would you allow me to interrupt you.*

"Later on, when we were waiting endlessly to see the doctor, Pol and I really talked as we never had before. I think the defenses she had so carefully built around herself for decades were eroding in the face of the oncoming mania. I realized that she had in all likelihood been depressed for a very, very long time."

It was an interminable wait and I spent my time making endless phone calls, *"perfectly orchestrated conversations on all four phones,"* according to my friend.

5

Once I was called in to the doctor, I made very sure Louisa came with me – giving evidence of my instinctive fear of being locked up. They couldn't do it if we were together, could they?

"Why are you asking me all these silly questions?" I asked the ER psychiatrist, who finally sent me off with a prescription for Lithium and an admonition to set up additional psychiatric consultation. I believe now that the Lithium saved me from escalating into a full-blown episode. At the time I totally rejected the idea that there was anything wrong, though being a good little girl, I dutifully took the medication and set up the psychiatric appointments.

Our meetings were just as inconsequential as the one at the hospital. The psychiatrist treated me like a cipher – an example of the illness rather than as an individual. I felt every appointment was an insult to my intelligence and am still appalled at what little effort he put into his "treatment" of me.

Perhaps I might have been in some last vestige of the almost manic state I'd reached, or perhaps it was just naivete, but I'd thought we could be friends, though I had no respect for his psychiatric acuity. I gave him a pot for his office and one for his wife – perfectly normal behavior for a lousy businesswoman who had always much preferred giving away her pottery than selling it. I've always wished I'd taken them back.

Horrified at this doctor's insensitivity, his rote responses, inattention, and the excessive amount I was paying him for what were eminently useless sessions, I cancelled the visits after a few months and at some point after that gave up the Lithium. I was still completely convinced the spell had just been due to over-work and exhaustion.

The psychiatrist's lack of interest and that of so many others of the medical profession in dealing with my illness have had vast repercussions for me and my family and set up the probability of other manic episodes, often purely through inattention. Those victims of mental disorders who have found decent psychiatrists, psycho-pharmacologists or therapists are the lucky (and rare) ones.

I had always been able to count on my body for terrific physical health, so (irresponsibly as I know now) my doctors' visits were erratic and for various reasons records did not follow me from one office to the next. I was busy, I didn't bother to seek good medical attention – the normal, awful reality of the millions of us who deny that we have any mental disorder whatsoever.

Chapter Two:

The Trip: Setting the Stage

Aquilon
Coming from your
pure white wall
I'm awed
longing
sad
You speak to my
sensuous soul.

The depth of Don's emotion towards our beautiful, canoe-sterned 50-year old wooden boat Aquilon was perhaps always greater than mine – I could never quite relate to her length and bulk. But spotting her in Tortola in 1996 had taken both our breaths away and though we had a perfectly decent boat already, we moved heaven and earth (and many replaced frames and planks) to maintain and restore her.

In the spring of 1999, both of us having given up our respective businesses, we began to prepare for Don's dream. The proposal was for Don and a crew of three to sail Aquilon (a 45-foot sloop) from Martha's Vineyard to the island of Grenada -- a journey of perhaps three weeks – leave her securely anchored there off Hog Island overseen by the former owner of this lovely boat. Then Don and I would fly down in late September and begin the long sail home.

He was approaching 70, physically fit, fearless by nature, calm and secure. As he'd recently retired, he felt he needed this adventure while he was still healthy and strong. With a few passages on sailboats to the Caribbean under his belt, a working knowledge of GPS, radar, single-sideband radio transmissions, an intimate understanding of Aquilon and her structure, and years of ownership of 30-38 foot fishing boats, Don had every reason to feel capable of doing a seven-month trip.

My sailing background was entirely different – summers spent on Martha's Vineyard, swimming at three, sailing at four, racing at five. I learned the hard way – in massively heavy 12-foot wooden "dogboats" – unwieldy, lumbering craft. It was a wonderful, tough way to learn skills and feel comfortable on a boat. Capsizing was often the norm and we loved it.

We finally graduated into "15s" – 15 feet at the waterline, 21 feet overall. That size remains about perfect for me, for my self confidence and control. The cut of the sails, the heeling of the boat, learning to play the sails skillfully to achieve optimum speed – all part and parcel of my youth. Truly coming to grips with a vessel more than double that size and many times its weight turned out to be impossible, though neither Don nor I wanted to admit it.

The plan went forward. We would sail the boat back from Grenada together, slowly and beautifully, cruising along when the winds and weather were perfect. We would anchor for days and steep ourselves in island history, take endless hikes of exploration, read all the books we'd ever wanted to read, swim and snorkel and become incredibly lithe and strong. Our visions were of translucent blue waters, dazzling sunsets (maybe even the green flash), sunny tropical days interspersed with the quirky, violent and blessedly brief Caribbean showers. Heaven.

We gradually began to eliminate the ties to our lives. For Don, the task was to take care of the thousands of details, especially readying the boat. For me, the details were the easy part. Most difficult was the prospect of letting go the newly-created opportunities for mediation after many years of training, learning and practice, adjusting to the prospect of no woman friends and no family. As a curious and friendly participant in the world of social interaction, my attitude towards the trip was less positive, but I was determined to help Don fulfill his dream.

Don and his crew delivered the boat safely to Grenada in June of 1999 and in late September we flew down and spent October in awestruck contemplation of our new life. Under orders from the insurance company, we could not sail past 12 degrees north until November first. And so the calm, dreamy days at anchor in Hog Island drifted by – marathon swims luxuriating in clean waters, beach cookouts with dozens of cruisers' children playing tag in the mangroves, bus trips and van rides all over this lush and mountainous island, endless games of Scrabble using the complicated Bequia rules.

We lived on Aquilon with no real agenda, though the strong Puritan ethic instilled in me by my father would not allow me to while away the days without something valuable to do – he would have been horrified by the frivolity of the whole trip. So I scrubbed the bottom with great fervor (too much, actually) to rid the boat of the "dreaded terredos," clever little boring tropical worms that have destroyed wooden hulls for centuries. But the month of October was almost totally restful, companionable and fun, and although the northward journey was our goal, we set off on November 1st with some regret.

And our dreams seemed to come true for a while – the harbors were welcoming, our explorations fascinating, markets teemed with gorgeous vegetables and exotic fruits, we visited with other cruisers we'd met along the way. Everything was going according to plan, except for the "boat boys" who rushed out to meet us at the entrance to harbors, ready to set our stern anchor or tie the boat to a palm tree or force us to hire them to watch the dinghy. Their attentions were frightening, given the prospect of holes bored in our wooden hull if we didn't comply and pay. We curtailed our visits to some islands because of them.

Our trip, and the lives of thousands of people in the Caribbean were drastically re-arranged by the arrival of a monstrous hurricane that November – past the normal hurricane season and, incredibly, arriving from the west with no warning. We were secure on three anchors in a mangrove hole in Martinique, but all the lovely places we had intended to visit up the chain were destroyed. The hurricane was the precursor of the Christmas winds – the expected heavy winds that normally go through January, but that year continued well into March – they were my downfall.

Fear of these strong winds stands out as the deepest emotional pitfall and problem I faced during these next months and, I believe, was a major contributor to my breakdown in June of 2000. For the most part, it was completely irrational (I knew this) – our boat was incredibly strong, built to cross oceans and climb high seas. Telling myself this did absolutely no good.

Unfortunately for me, the wind always came out of the southeast – our trip was almost entirely headed northwest, so we were usually running before the wind. The sails are both way out and the motion of rocking back and forth is set up and increases as the wind and waves increase. As a child, I had always been terrified of this point of sail. To this day, even on an afternoon of lazy social sailing, the prospect of setting up the rolling fills me with dread.

At its simplest denominator, my fear was that the boat would rock right over to one side or the other and would be unable to right itself. We would lose everything and probably our lives, as we were often way off land and sailing overnight when the difficult passages from island to island occurred. Actually, in considering my particular terror, I never carried the consequences that far – it was just this horrible feeling as the boat lurched from side to side – nothing our two combined weights could change. We would reef (shorten) the sails but nothing really helped. Needless to say, I couldn't help Don steer – I just huddled in the cockpit, looking straight ahead to avoid seeing the enormous waves high above the stern. My terror during those night passages was truly beyond description.

In addition to the fear, and perhaps exaggerating it, was my dreadful insomnia. A wire inside the steel mast banged noisily each night when we were at anchor and my sleeping hours were limited to three or maximum four. No one operates intelligently with as little sleep as I was getting.

"5:03 AM, January 16, Marigot, St. Martin's. What it's like to be in a huge wind – very very unpleasant. It is virtually impossible to sleep. First, there is so much noise – the wind itself howling in through the hatches, deafeningly loud. If you close up to lessen that particular noise, you can't breathe. The internal slapping of the halyard inside the mast. Tonight I've tried everything, and actually found the forward berths pretty comfortable, forwards and backwards, and there the mast racket lessens. BUT, then you have the anchor chain groaning and screeching as the boat bucks and snorts and the wind pushes it from side to side. The anchor clamor is an enormous banging, like a car accident, where the halyard noise is constant – bang bang bang bang quickly. And then of course we are rolling from side to side, sometimes ferociously. T.paper in the ears doesn't work. I doubt any means would work tonight.

"And these things always happen at night, it seems but this one may go on for another whole day and night. Being on deck tonight is wild – boats madly rocking in great disarray, none the same. Tonight even Don is awake – he's pretty good at sleeping through the halyard banging, the rolling. Not this time."

Erskine Childers wrote beautifully about a similar situation: "*Every loose article in the boat became audibly restless. Cans clinked, cupboards rattled, lockers uttered hollow groans. Small things sidled out of dark hiding-places, and danced grotesque drunken figures on the floor, like goblins in a haunted glade. The mast whined dolorously at every heel, and the centerboard hiccoughed and choked. Overhead another horde of demons seems to have been let loose. The deck and mast were conductors which magnified every sound and made the tap-tap of every rope's end resemble the blows of a hammer, and the slapping of the halyards against the mast the rattle of a Maxim gun. The whole tumult beat time to a rhythmical chorus which became maddening.*"

As the winds increased, anchors dragged and boats crashed into each other. Don valiantly went forward to begin the laborious work of hauling up our anchor so we could avoid these dangerous collisions. In trying to come up slowly to help him in his task, I could not keep the boat into the wind. Being unwilling and too terrified to give up when I failed, we almost rammed three boats. Luckily Don came back and put it in reverse – so much for my quick reactions in an emergency.

The situation deteriorated, but we were able to extricate the anchor at last, traverse the wild harbor safely and re-anchor outside the breakwater – not surrounded by other boats. What we didn't consider was that we were then in 10 feet of water and the surf (not swells, not waves, but *surf*) kept building, building. We would rise up and hover on top of the crest, hold our breaths until the boat came crashing down, shaking all its beams and timbers. The dinghy roamed madly back and forth behind us in the surf – losing that expensive piece of equipment would have been very bad, given our already slim budget. Don put out yet another anchor – minutes seemed like hours.

We finally decided this was more dangerous than trying to find a safe path through the boats in the harbor, so we worked our way painfully back through the seething anchorage, finally settling behind the breakwater. The next day we apologized to the captain whose boat we had almost sideswiped. He graciously accepted our apology, telling us *"I very nearly crashed into two boats yesterday myself and I learned that the winds reached 70 miles an hour. That enormous tanker has gone aground on the other side of the breakwater."*

I picked up my journal the next day. "This is not what we bargained for or even could have imagined. My fears, described above a little, pale in comparison with the last 24 hours. Don, the stoic, just got through and didn't even really want to talk about it. I've been in tears or hysterical all day. Our exhaustion is deep. Sleepless night plus all that emotional strain of this horrible day. I guess it's critical to remember that we did indeed live through this (though we haven't yet, it's night and the winds are still howling around us). Maybe things can't get worse. It surely does make you wonder what the hell you're doing here."

My fear grew over these months, with incidents like this one and with the dreaded dark and terrifying passages. But eventually our adventure was over – two others sailed Aquilon home from the Bahamas. It would be a huge understatement to say that our return was a disappointment. We were dispensable, life had gone on just fine without us. Remarks like, *"I can't keep track of you, you two are never here."*

Two of my best friends were so involved in a conversation about a local drama concerning one of them that they hardly said hello. My hurt was tremendous and on top of all the personal stuff, many of the mediation jobs for which I had trained and worked towards for years had been taken on by people I had trained myself. My feeling of dislocation was complete. I had become an absentee landlord of my life.

And so we went back to Maine in June of 2000, having rented our home on Cape Cod.

As Patty Duke said before a breakdown, *"The recipe was perfect. Start with genetics, add a lot of loss and a lot of turmoil. What you end up with is a classic manic depressive."* I think my recipe was perfect too.

Chapter Three:

My First Major Episode in 2000

Where's the fairness –
in a day I've become
extinct
sidelined to the bench
no more need to feed the love
of kindred thoughts –
What's sad is
she seems to mean it.
Does she really know?

"Don, why shouldn't I throw my clothes down the stairs? Obviously it's the best way to clean out the closet and all the stuff I have. You always tell me to get rid of my clothes, why would you wonder at all what I'm doing?"

And later, "We've always agreed with each other that television doesn't belong in our special old farmhouse, so it was really time I threw it out the window. It was a lot easier than carrying it down the stairs. You know my old friend Don Hendrie took care of his kids' bad tv watching habits that way, so I thought I'd just follow his lead. I absolutely can't figure out why you don't understand it was the best thing to do."

These two examples of my mounting mania occurred right before the Brooksville, Maine annual fundraiser for the library, which has such a small budget that it can only survive with the aid of such events -- this one was a tour of some wonderful local gardens. I felt especially articulate, charming and intelligent as I toured the various locales and was even invited to dinner at a virtual stranger's home later on that week. The next day, I visited a garden I'd missed at the home of someone I'd just met but whom I liked a great deal and thought might become a friend.

I stayed and stayed, chatting happily and admiring her gardens, only wondering after a while why her husband was sitting by the garage with his dog, rather than taking it for a walk. She eventually went into the house, pleading the need to make dinner. I just waited there happily, circling the house, sure she'd come back out of the kitchen to talk. In all likelihood, she was terrified I would break in to see her, but I was having an extraordinarily good time just being there. It absolutely never occurred to me that she didn't feel the same way. Eventually, her husband reached Don, who came to get me. (The next summer, I was so deeply ashamed that I avoided her, but now, years later, we are gradually becoming good friends.)

Life was perfect as I drove back to the house, Don

having driven on ahead, confused and concerned, as were all our friends. I was so pleased, but not at all surprised, that even with no phone in the car, I could talk to people I knew all over the country. They talked, I answered— who knows what we talked about. I knew I had never been in such a good mood.

I arrived very happily at the town dock, sat looking merrily at the stars, talking to myself a mile a minute. There seemed to be so much to say. Never had I been filled with so much complete joy. It was so wonderful having extensive conversations with my long-deceased parents, whom I had adored. Most of my life's enduring problems were getting important recognition from the heavens and were resolved. Even the worst one, my childlessness, became a non-issue that night. Of course no one could have two birth mothers – so my goddaughters and my niece and nephew just lucked out and landed with a second, just as important mother: me. What a relief to reach that conclusion. How sad that my epiphany on this score and others disappeared with the mania.

As an episode escalates, manic depressives are not willing to give up the incredible feelings of creativity, fast-flowing ideas, artistic solutions to life's challenges and problems. The idea of dulling the brain with medication is anathema to us, but the tragedy is that the mania spills out over the edge. John Custance hoped and believed that his *"abnormal experiences,"* which he desperately did not want to lose, could be controlled. He felt that a physician's duty was to explain to a patient what was in fact realizable and what is not, and then he could learn to adapt his abnormality to the conditions of the world.

How I wish those experiences could in fact be controlled, that my "epiphanies" (now I can't bear that word, given its implications for my manic states of mind) were still a part of me – some of course were nonsense, however some were glorious. What I especially miss of the mania is the extraordinary loss of the Watcher – the critical observer who has analyzed and harshly judged my every move, my every word, since my early twenties. During my manic states, the Watcher disappeared and with it my self-consciousness. I was treated to the awesome marriage of my intellect and my soul. I rejoiced, I danced and sang, I was fiercely intelligent and clever in social interactions. I especially didn't care if people liked me. I figured things out – all without second-guessing, self-observation, and self-critique. Perhaps most people live without the Watcher – how I envy them.

(nB: When I wrote these last words in 2007, I ended the paragraph, "But there is no choice: I cannot survive another episode." And since then there has indeed been another which I did survive, but it is such a tragic disappointment for me that the illness is still so much a part of my life.)

Evidence mounted quickly in the minds of friends, neighbors and Don that there was something seriously amiss – my constant talk, hysterical laughter at my own jokes, a complete disdain for food or sleep. Don wrote: *"The onset of Pol's erratic behavior was destabilizing, threatening the status quo that I had come to accept. Normally fun, gregarious, outgoing and enthusiastic suddenly going overboard. What can I do? Who can help? In a way it was a tornado bearing square upon you. You stand mesmerized and incapable watching."*

Just a night
then another day —
this could go on —
it does —
of anguish wanting surcease
Do you feel it too
or are you too enthralled
by your new
essence
that mortals leave you cold.

He gathered a crew of people I trusted in our driveway and somehow got me into a car, protesting all the way, most concerned about our new puppy, Pascal. My threat to throw a large rock from the campfire pit through the glass slider on the front porch was probably what got me admitted to the Emergency Room, as I was now potentially a danger to myself or to others.

This visit led rather dramatically to a hospitalization in another locale, and I wrote the following a few days later. (It interests me that at least as a descriptive piece, it's pretty clear and lucid.)

"I was told I was to have something to calm me down (OK with me). But when I heard it was to be a shot, I realized I was terrified of having a shot. I asked if it could be in pill form, they said absolutely not. It turned out to be Haldol, a medication which had done very strange things like tics to my sister's mouth for years. I had no objection to anything except the fact of its being a shot. Therewith started the whole thing.

"I couldn't bear the idea and fought against it, first with words then with my body when large men began to appear. At some point they tied me down. The nurse who'd been so insistent (and maybe by now had given me the shot) started taking my temperature with the ear thermometer. It hurt a great deal, I told her, and pled with her not to do it, but she kept viciously stabbing at my ears, first one then the other. It hurt a lot. Again, why couldn't they do it the time-honored way of sticking it in my mouth? I figure she was mad at me for making it so hard for her. So she kept taking my blood pressure, gave me some Valium. I guess they were waiting for me to calm down and stop fighting with them. Why should I have, when these happenings were going on? So there were lots of thug types there to get me on a stretcher to go somewhere. I kept resisting and of course made it all worse.

"So I get all strapped down and wheeled out to an ambulance. As the stretcher bumps up into the ambulance, I realize I desperately need to go to the bathroom -- it had been hours. I ask if we can go back in and the two men say, *"No, you have to wait til we get there. It's only about an hour away."* I'm in agony the whole trip, begging them to at least tip the stretcher up so maybe I could pee somehow. But I'm very tightly strapped in, no way could anyone do it under these circumstances.

"We get to the hospital and there is a nurse there saying to me, *"Oh, you have been behaving so badly. So very, very badly."* I beg over and over to go to the bathroom, no go. There is a man guarding the room after she leaves, I beg him to get me help. Every once in a while he desultorily calls for someone. Meanwhile, I'm in agony. There is no excuse for this. I would have just gone in the bed, but I was too tightly tied down. Finally, after what must have been an hour, I am allowed to use a bedpan. The nurse is so horrible to me, frowning at me, telling me how bad I am. So I drop the full bedpan off the bed (and of course get nastily chastised for it) and feel a little better and a bit gleeful.

"At some point this nurse and three guys come in and say I'm going to be undressed. I beg them not to touch my necklaces, they rip them off and break the clasps on both. The nurse tugs my tights off brusquely. The worst thug, with these huge arms, is hurting me a lot, holding on to my right arm in which the other hospital had left the i.v. still inserted. He pulls at it and it's all black and blue thereafter. Then he tries to pull off my bracelet – meanwhile I keep asking, "Why can't I do this?" It doesn't come easily at all, finally it gets manhandled off and I still have a bruise where it bled. The worst part of all this is that this particular man seemed to be taking such perverse pleasure in hurting me, making me cry. It was totally infuriating but they finally got me undressed and then God knows what happened next."

Perhaps one should feel compassion for those holding such unsatisfying and probably demoralizing jobs, but I can't find it in me. There seems to be nothing forgivable about these inhumane acts and others that came up later on. The incident I just described was certainly the most brutal in all my hospital stays – for the most part, staffers were just insensitive, nasty and short-tempered.

And so it began, this first hospitalization. Don, who was faithfully visiting every day, wrote that: *"The insides and operation of a psychiatric hospital are numbing. They have her. You have lost her. What are they doing? Is there an end to this or is normalcy gone – whatever that may be. You are losing control of things that you value. Your wife, your life. It started taking on a substance of a monster I didn't want in our life. Friends, advice, doctors, medication. The return to "normalcy became tentative. Life had become warped by this debilitating disease, as I was learning it was."*

"I could never have imagined what real incarceration would be like," I noted. "I still reach to open doors, only to be rebuffed by the fiercely locked steel door – just another impediment to my freedom. I never appreciated freedom, as it was totally taken for granted. Here I can only go to the bathroom, my bedroom and the rec room without a pass or with an escort. I suppose the staff is used to it. Do they go home and appreciate just reaching and opening a door? How long will I notice the ability to let myself in and out, I wonder, after I'm sprung?"

Every day in the hospital was "monumentally frustrating," and I longed for my freedom, but "I will survive. One thing imprisonment does is level the playing field. We're all equals in this institution, but some of us don't mind being here – life is too complicated on the outside, they have virtually nowhere to go. They might succeed in killing themselves if they go out."

I took notes on some of the patients. "The majority of people are depressed, several suicidal. One Penobscot Indian just came in: overdose, very sorry he didn't manage to kill himself. He is a totally gorgeous young man, 27 years old. Robin, an unbelievably gifted artist and very, very bright, had been raped and battered by her father, while her mother just stayed in denial and continues to support her husband. But amazingly enough, Robin is funny. She is unabashedly gay and constantly talks about it, she longs for a long-term relationship, has no home to go to. She checked herself in because she couldn't stop trying to commit suicide.

"Some substance abuse, though not much. Jason, the wiseacre, doesn't know when to stop teasing, but he's very young. Pat's mother put him in here, supposedly because he stopped eating for two days. Came back from a weekend pass completely catatonic, having peroxided his hair – looks horrible. And Kelly, a large male who wants to be a woman, with huge glasses, stringy gray hair, cries a lot, suddenly decides 'she' likes you and envelops you in a huge, not very welcome bear hug. I don't understand her at all, but as usual am pleased we are friends.

"And Ana, my roommate – raped, beaten, smothered by her father from age 2, rickets from her mother's malnutrition leaving her with virtually no knee on one leg, very weak one on the other. Raped by her brother and gave birth to twins. Two other sets of twins, all aborted somehow. Now almost blind, catheterized constantly so she wears diapers." (Don was barely able to prevent my wildly cheerful and enthusiastic gift of a $700 rent check to Ana, who was in grave financial trouble.)

"And Dale, depressed, despondent over her mother's death, usually works at Shop and Save. Quiet, flat voice and no affect. And lots of others, including a new, rather bizarre creature named Candance – she's Cherokee. Most sentences have fu--ing in them, it gets really old and annoying. I feel no kindness towards her at all, she's creating huge havoc on the ward, but she is so crazy you can't torment her back, as Jason does. There are others and it's easy to get their stories being here with them. In the beginning no one talked to each other. I think I started the communication piece of this and got the group talking."

I tried to describe the physical plant: "the usual gray/green walls, twin-bed quarters, a common room with old movie magazines, a television, people shuffling around looking vacant. But outside we're surrounded by quite pretty land and yesterday we came upon a fabulously lush garden box with hugely verdant leaves on the tomato plants, zillions of flowers and vines of cucumbers cascading down the wall. We'll plagiarize the idea for sure. The teepees for the beans are good, the straw keeping down the weeds. It's so lush and yummy. Foot-high basil ready for pesto or salad dressing." It's the only good thing I can remember about this first hospitalization – actually about any of them.

Others have eloquently described the inanity, the non-therapeutic environment of a typical mental hospital.

There is usually virtually nothing to do besides useless group sessions. Discussions with the ward psychiatrists are no more fruitful nor even interesting. "The amazing thing is there is no therapy. This is just a holding tank for us fish. Just a place to use drugs and calm people down, then eventually shoot them out somewhere."

There was only an unpredictable, 15-minute walk on weekday mornings, nothing on weekends. "Good Lord," I noted, "no wonder my legs have turned to spaghetti. But more importantly, there are very disturbed, suicidal people in here and for them to release some sort of tension is imperative. Probably they'd say it's how many staff members are required for an outdoor walk. They give zillions of cigarette breaks, but no exercise. Yikes."

My recollections of the staff are negative across the board: "They're totally unapproachable, they never introduce themselves nor do they ever look at you. I tromp up and down the endless halls, no one even gives me a side glance. Going up to the staff window is a humiliating experience, as they are usually rude and distant: *What do you want **this** time?*" Another patient said to me, *"They obviously aren't doing anything else, so why can't they be nice to us? They won't even bother to come to the window.'"*

The best and worst example from that same note: "Joanne, sitting alone in medication room, only staffer on duty, it's 1:30 AM. I go past and say, 'I'm sorry, I forgot your name.' She finally looks at me and says, *'Joanne.'* I disappear, reappear about ½ hour later, say something frivolous, she looks down, down. Finally I say, 'Well, it's really nice when someone looks at you when you speak to them so you know they've heard what you said.' She not only doesn't look at me, she looks farther away. I stand there aghast for a minute or so, then go back to my room, fuming."

I hope there was more method to this staff's madness. Another blatant example of what I considered their insensitivity stands out. There was a young patient, Richard, a seemingly retarded 29-year old, almost illiterate but a gifted sketcher. Too much stress at home had led him into foster care, now he just wanted to have a job and a dog. As he was having some sort of epileptic seizure, I put my arm around his shoulder and my hand between his neck and other shoulder. I thought a caring hand was worth a lot during this hard time – his head just kept bobbing and bobbing and he said this made him feel better. *"Stop it, take your hands off him,"* yelled the staffer who pushed me away. Who knew the rules about touching, I wondered. So much for trying to be kind.

I reflected in my notes that "It would be so very simple to introduce oneself (a staff member) to new people, say we're here to help, let us know how we can do this. A new person is just thrown in here, thrown to the wolves. No one makes an effort to teach any rules, consequently I make hordes of mistakes. But it would be so easy."

Getting into trouble was what I did best, mostly through ignorance of the rules. Logic alone made it clear to me that simple explanations about times for walking, telephone use, cigarette breaks, the pass system could be given with no difficulty at the morning "discussions." Instead, there was nothing. Eventually, after asking for days why my requests for passes were turned down, I was finally told, *"You are much too intrusive and you just want to know too many things. Why don't you stop asking so many questions and just sit down and be quiet like the other patients?"*

At least the ward psychiatrist was polite, though it was difficult to respect her acuity when our conversations began and continued with, *"Did you sleep well? Did you go for a walk this morning?"* Nothing more important than that, no therapy, no thoughtful discussions, ever. I wrote her a letter, pleading to be released to see my nephew and his family, who had driven 10 hours to visit with us.

"I just need to get back into my world. I figure I have already paid my dues here, I go to every group I can, I've gotten the whole ward to open up to me and to each other in a way that was not happening when I came in. Now they are actually conversing with each other during breaks, in the dining room. This was not true until I broke the silence barrier. For days until I dared to talk with a few of them, I thought they were total zombies, so I concentrated on group dynamics. It worked, and I immodestly know I take a great deal of credit for it. This will be a much more silent and unhappy place when I go, of that I can be sure.

"This place is negating the positive aspects of my personality. I try to do good things and they are put down. I get enthusiastic about something and I am classified as manic. I walk around more than other people and I am classified as manic. I try to clean up the disgusting cigarette area (deadhead flowers, weed, rake up butts, water plants) and I'm again manic in the eyes of the staff. Did you ever think that I do all these things because I am bored here from lack of constructive activity and that cleaning is a coping strategy in an attempt to ward off that boredom?

"I try to teach my roommate to be thoughtful and point out to her that she's been hogging the phone for an hour and someone else needs to make a more important call, I get yelled at, then in fun I throw a small plastic bottle in the corner of the room where she is sitting (not at her) and I am FORCED to take an Ativan. Later I'm told I didn't have to take it. Well, when you have a very large staff member screaming at you from 3 inches away and you've always been an obedient child, you damn well take the Ativan. Then yesterday I was exhausted, tearful, slept most of the afternoon and went to bed early, all because of the damn pill, I realize.

"So what more can I do to be released????? I do my very, very best here, I've made lots of friends, I've cleaned up the TV room, the gardens, the bookcases in the rec room." Of course there was no response to this plea, no discussion with the doctor – only a final release from the hospital before I was to be sent before a judge.

Most importantly, the medications **had** calmed me down, the mania had disappeared, but there just has to be a way to help patients in my position have one or two useful moments in a hospital, to learn even one thing, instead of what in my case were almost two completely wasted weeks.

The medication had restored my balance and I was sent clear-headed back out into my world. Though I'd lost my waitressing job at the small restaurant in our town and I worried desperately about the people who had been disturbed by my peculiar behavior, I believe the rest of the summer was all right. No depression, in other words, unlike the years later when it came on with a vengeance.

Chapter Four:

Denial and Its Consequences in 2003

No one wants to believe he has any kind of life-long, often life-threatening illness, but it is a special disaster for a manic depressive to deny his disease and refuse help. Denial is so predictable and so prevalent among us. It leads to all kinds of horror: more hospitalizations, violence, suicide. Fifteen percent of manic depressives succeed in committing suicide, but when they hurt themselves or others, it is almost always due to giving up their medications. Denial goes hand in hand with an insistence on assuming and retaining control over oneself, just when one is incapable of it.

I had completely eradicated the reality of the short episode in 1994, and though the hospital weeks in 2000 represented some harsh truths, I assured myself and everyone else that the experience was "one of a kind, not to be repeated." Having lived with my sister, my husband and a close friend through bouts of mania, I was sure I had a handle on it and understood the nature of the disease better than anyone. My doctor left town, the records disappeared, I gradually stopped taking the medication and forgot about the whole thing. Don had no reason to think I wasn't taking it. My irresponsibility came back to bite me in early June.

This time, the great cheer, the sleeplessness, the starvation were accompanied by waves of anger towards some members of our family. Irritability is one of the hallmarks of mania and only increases as the episode deteriorates. (The last time I'd felt so angry was in April of 2000, a little less than two months before my first real episode. When I realized we were throwing in the towel, having others sail the boat home, I was horrified and furious -- here we finally were in our ultimate gorgeous place – Georgetown, Great Exuma, the Bahamas. I raged at Don for giving up on this adventure before it was over, for his overly careful behavior on the boat which had often prevented us from seeing much of the islands we were visiting. "Your lack of lightheartedness in general infuriates me and I hate ending it feeling this way. I hate these vast feelings of anger and fury that have been plaguing me.")

"Aha," I wrote to myself three years later, "a long honest letter demanding honesty from the family will do the trick. I'll take Pascal out for a long walk while they read it and if they won't talk sincerely and deal with this problem, I don't want to have anything to do with them, including Don, ever again." I carefully equipped myself with tools for the drive back to the Cape from Maine: tape recorder, yellow pads, pens, cigarettes. I set off, ready to compose this critical tome. It was early June, 2003.

I noticed and applauded how carefully I was driving. First, I made some notes on the pad, pulling it back and forth from the other seat until I realized I could leave it in my lap – I laughed about that for a while. I wrote down the exact hour and minutes when I added phrases to the letter – 5:02, 5:19, etc. Smoking furiously, I kept losing matches and cigarettes in the car.

Things I could do got narrowed down: first I could write, light a cigarette, listen to the radio and drive at the same time. Then only smoke, listen and drive. Then listen and drive. Then the radio had to be turned off. My voyage downhill. With great amusement I noted that I should send my scribblings to someone as an example of bipolar thinking.

At a rest stop about three hours along my journey, I ran into a lovely painter whom we knew a bit and whose work we admired. She was deluged with my overwhelming good will, chatter, verbose explanations of euphoria and startling epiphanies. How terrifying it was for her, but as usual, I thought I was completely charming. She told me later, *"I didn't think I could ever extricate myself and get back on the road."* Finally, we went on our respective ways and I returned safely to the Cape, notes and tapes in hand.

My wonderful good cheer proceeded side by side with frustration at being misunderstood, my great thoughts being undervalued, especially by Don. I wrote him a letter which I think makes sense, but just the fact that I wrote it out could be seen as another sign of my falling apart.

"Don, I love you. We have been together 25 years, for better or worse. I have reached a point in my life where I need you to listen – not all the time – with an open heart and mind. It may be quick and dirty, it may take all day. But if we are to spend the rest of our lives together, I cannot continue to rely on my close women friends to care and to empathize and to listen. You're a great listener when you try – I guess I want it 100%, or at least to set a date when I truly have your attention." I thought my desperate need to be listened to was a legitimate demand, but it's extremely doubtful I was doing any listening myself.

Don was fighting hard to understand and counteract the mania, and this time it was made even more intolerable by my undiluted anger.

Where has she gone
I do not know
I think she makes her home aloft
somewhere
in wild flights of fantasy
beyond my ken
I try to look, to see, to understand
but in my heart it's useless –
I know she doesn't want me there.

One day after a night I'd spent loudly muttering, singing, clattering around the house on the Cape so that neither my sister Harriet nor Don could sleep at all, he refused to let me drive the car. I was furious, ran to the neighbor's and got a ride to town. Much to my complete amazement, a man living next to the grocery store wouldn't let me in to use his phone. I couldn't believe it – Eastham, our small, safe town? I must have frightened him badly.

Suddenly I was confronted with the police, Don and Harriet, who coaxed me across the street to the fire department where they took my blood pressure and asked me some questions. Harriet told me later, *"You were so friendly, so articulate, so interested in the men's families and their lives – just the picture of a lovely, curious and polite woman."* In fact, it was the picture of a very smart and manipulative manic depressive well along on her way out of control.

My memory of events is sketchy here, but apparently Don and Harriet felt somewhat secure that I was all right and returned to Maine and the Vineyard. I wasn't, by any means, and I think now that the most painful part of writing this account was my recent discovery of some outrageously manic notes written on an entire yellow pad as I drove crazily to see my cousin, who lives about an hour from our home on the Cape.

The notes were all part of a letter I was trying to write her, assuring her of my and my family's eternal love for her. The letter begins: "Hi Kat. I love you SO MUCH. MADLY." It was way before dawn as I drove along, I planned to sleep in her living room, wake her up with this marvelous letter and introduce her to Pascal. As before, I carefully made note of the very specific hour and minute of each new addition.

"I HEAR THE BIRDS!! I know PASCAL HEARD ME. She UNDERSTANDS EVERYTHING I say. Every single word." I was so thrilled by this and wanted to tell Harriet: "Hat, I instantly thought of Google. You'd look me up as a phenomenon right away." We went around a rotary several times and headed north, the wrong direction, and stopped behind a gas station. "I realized Pascal was only (probably) hearing her name. ha...ha. 3 minutes of disappointment. Hat, there go the billions."

We kept going. "Anyway, time to drive again. The modern miracle and her consort." The driving mistakes I kept making struck me as hysterically funny and I made careful notes of exactly when I burst out laughing again. Dozens of miracles (which were assuredly nonsense) were going on in my head and it was critical that they be circled in my notes. I wasn't allowed to speak out loud without the circles, or the miracles would disappear. "FINAL PROOF FOR THE WORLD." I wonder what that was.

Having been lost for what might have been hours, I surprised myself by recognizing a beautiful old building where a friend of mine worked. It was around 5:00 AM. Pascal chased the ball merrily up and down the stone steps while I struggled to write my friend a letter – I'm not sure if I ever completed it. I was laughing and laughing, writing and re-writing, wishing I had some carbon paper, wondering how often I'd have to do it before it looked all right. I've never asked that poor girl about it – I haven't seen her and I'm too ashamed. "How can I ever finish this? It's so hard to keep remembering to circle the miracles. At least I am sure I spoke normally with that young jogger."

It seems, according to my family, that I never got to my cousin's. My last note reads, "After all this time I am exhausted but driving safely."

Even in all the crazy notes I found and some of which I have related, I thought I was "always conscious when writing to be very clear so no one can doubt my head is screwed on right. It is so awful to be so happy, thoughtful, etc., and keep worrying it indicates a manic attack." So there it was that year: an awareness and a denial mixed together. Clearly I couldn't convince myself I was all right and I especially failed in convincing others.

Somehow I ended up in the *only* really worthwhile mental treatment program that I've experienced anywhere: the Outpatient Psych Program in the hospital on the Cape. There were accessible, bright staff members offering small workshops on manic depression and different types of mental illness, some excellent videos – generally a good, educational and respectful atmosphere. Luckily, I kept their flyers and my notes from these three days.

The stress throughout the workshop was on understanding and compassion. "Mental illness is NOT A CHARACTER FLAW," I wrote proudly in huge letters. There were discussions of depression and the seduction of mania, the manic depressive's unwillingness to give up his creativity, his uniqueness. The staff explained the causes which I understand so much better now: chemical imbalance, genetics, extreme crises, loss, subsequent vulnerability. It felt so wonderful finally to be among intelligent people who would talk about all this and I felt I had a great deal to contribute. I was calm and appreciative and "I had myself back."

One workshop spoke of families, how they should recognize there is a problem, that the patient in denying the illness has lost his objectivity. How they should let the patients know they care, encourage them to get help, stand by them, be strong, but not take responsibility for them. That last is usually too difficult for families.

Another group dealt with coping strategies and goals for the patients themselves: "taking responsibility for own medication, therapy, watching for signs (e.g. anger, erratic behavior), keeping a mood journal, preparing for relapse, sharing the signals, talking with friends and going over cues, avoiding triggering situations (major life changes, problems in living, losses), having fun, laughing, communicating with the doctor, reaching out for support." All of this was presented in an informal, supportive way, and it felt great. And it's exactly the information anyone with a manic history or manic predisposition should have.

I happily made a list of the 10 things I was grateful for: "Love of friends, love of family, good health, good mind, good listening skills (improving), wonderful parents and education, successful pottery business, knowing Robert Kennedy, loss of this huge depression, PASCAL." The whole tone of the workshop was upbeat and engaging – we were being trained to understand our illness in a positive way. They tried to teach us to consider the positive parts of our lives as well as to help us with skills for tolerating painful events and emotions when we can't make things better right away.

The presenters encouraged us to make a chart of the facts and stresses before or during episodes. My chart below would be completely typical of other victims of this illness, but the specific details would differ.

1994	2000	2003	
X	X	X	decreased appetite, sleeplessness
X			recent loss of Mahzie (my mother)
	X		loss of Aunt Pol, Woofie (a very close friend), Tasha, my dog
	X	X	loss of friends and life as I knew it
X	X	X	racing thoughts
		X	irritability, anxiety
	X		paralyzing fear and insomnia

X	X	X	disorganized thinking
		X	decreased attention span
		X	poor concentration
		X	unable to cope with minor stresses
		X	hyper-organized, compulsive

The workshop ended on a Friday and a very impressive psychiatrist gave me a prescription for a strong anti-psychotic medication. I was expected back on the unit on Monday and I was looking forward to more participation in the program. This was not to be. I didn't fill the prescription, deciding to do it later in the day on Saturday after I'd cleaned the houses we rented. It was more convenient to do it on the way to a birthday party for my close friend Mykee's husband, Bill.

"You can't come in the house," the newly-arrived tenant said firmly, to my complete surprise. "If you'll just wait ten minutes, I can finish the vacuuming," I replied – no luck. He continued to bar the door. I couldn't understand why this man seemed so terribly angry, as I'd always had a great relationship with his wife and was being most agreeable. So what if I was a little delayed with the cleaning? I was positive I'd done no wrong, I was so happy, things were going so well. Apparently

I scared the wits out of them, but as usual I can only imagine how frightening my behavior was.

Who knows what occupied me for so long that I was four hours late to Bill's birthday party – the last guests were on their way out the door. I did ask someone to fill the prescription at an all-night drugstore – it didn't materialize and would probably have been too late by then. Reportedly, I drank a lot of wine and the hosts finally went to bed. I roamed all around the house, kept drinking, made a mess of the kitchen and in the end went to my car to call my friend Betsy way after midnight. Apparently the conversation went on for hours. At some point, I fell asleep out there in the yard.

(Manic depressives are known to spend hours and hours on the phone every day and night. As Robert Lowell wrote in 1964, *"I want to apologize for plaguing you with so many telephone calls last November and December. When the 'enthusiasm' is coming on me it is accompanied by a feverish reaching to my friends. After it's over I wince and wither."* My inclination was the same – just calling Information two years later cost over $200 one month. I can't even bear to record the amount of money spent on phone bills, expensive changes in cell phone services to meet my growing requirements, and loss of the phones themselves.)

Mykee found me asleep in the car in the morning, door open, battery dead. The family was all gathering for a Father's Day feast and post-birthday celebration. Unfortunately, I had joyfully fed the better part of their dinner to Pascal the night before. Mykee was forced to spend four hours getting me to a drugstore and run interference between me and the pharmacist, *"as you had become so belligerent and rude."* Finally, my sister came and took over. I was hospitalized, in a *"hypomanic state of agitation, anger and irritability."*

According to hospital notes, I was *"hyper-verbal, tangential, her thought content is a word salad."* My *"insight, judgment and impulse control"* were non-existent at the time of my admission – of course I, on the other hand, thought I was making perfect sense and couldn't for the life of me figure out why I was there. Papers were filed for a commitment after I demanded to leave the hospital, but before the court hearing, I agreed to sign in with a specific discharge date planned – 12 days later. The medication I had been neglecting to take was re-prescribed in addition to the very strong anti-psychotic I should have taken earlier.

As before, I was terribly angry to be there: "The main problem is I was not informed that as a voluntary patient I was to be locked in. NO ONE informed me. This is intolerable. I JUST WANT to be free." As before, I considered myself a model of manners and the staff, "gratuitously rude." I remember requesting a staff member to smile at me; his response was: *"I believe I smiled at you when you arrived."*

I honestly don't know if this staff was particularly nasty to the patients or not. As I didn't have my tape recorder nor my computer and therefore made no notes, this hospitalization is lost in my memory. Besides the quotes above, all I really remember is being transported in restraints in an ambulance the 200 yards from the hospital to its Psych Unit. It seemed ridiculous at the time. It still does.

Even though I hardly recollect that she was there at all, my friend Marcia recalls two visits with me which she describes as, *"colorless, lacking in visual reassurance that there was a world outside the double doors. We met in the dining room, which also serves as the community room. Polly was ever the gracious hostess, greeting me and the other patients, introducing us as though we were all guests at her bed and breakfast, or patrons of her pottery shop, or potential voters for her national candidate – it was an unusual experience for me."*

"I could only listen as she spoke of how stupid the personnel were and how poorly they treated these other patients or how often she had to clean the community area. I reminded myself that her lack of self assessment is an exquisitely frustrating part of mental illness.

"I was moved to doubtful hope for Polly's healing, since other people I had visited had gone into integrated lives full of family and work and joy. Perhaps the same could happen for her. I knew my friend. Her considerable intelligence, her passion, her education, the love she attracted from us all could heal. Would it?

"When I was able to visit Pol again a few days later, I was surprised. The eager friend who greeted me seemed a lot closer to the woman I knew outside the hospital. 'Great news,' she said, 'We can go for a walk.' *Outside?* I asked. "Oh yes, I'm so excited," she replied. *For the first time in my experience with Polly's disease, I felt fear. Was I to be*

47

expected to care for my tall friend through traffic and crowds of downtown Hyannis? What if she decided she would like to thumb home or hop a bus? Or entertain the masses on a soapbox of political science? I swallowed my fear and turned it over to the vision of wellness I had hoped for. Maybe it had arrived and just maybe the psychiatric staff knew what they were doing in allowing this freedom. Maybe Polly was in charge of her own safety and not me.

"Off we went and all was going well for the first block until Pol announced she was going to buy cigarettes. The friend I knew did not smoke. Again the fear…did the staff approve? I said I would not buy them for her, but would wait while she executed this little self-destructive act. Out she came from a CVS and happily lit up. At least we returned safely to the hospital and she resumed her restricted life."

The amazing truth is that neither my past close relationship with manic depressives, the experience in 2000, nor the intense, excellent workshop a few weeks earlier had persuaded me that I had the illness and that in all likelihood it would re-appear. And yet it did, two years later.

Chapter Five:

Reason No Longer Controls the Chariot

A psychiatric nurse really did a number on me in 2005, taking me off my bi-polar medication. *"Since I really doubt that you are a manic depressive,"* she averred, *"and your Depakote level is so low, let's try Lamictal. The only side effect of it is a rash, and if it develops, stop it immediately and call me. I think this will help with your depression."*

The change in medication happened toward the end of February and we planned to see each other once a month. As it turns out, administering this medication is supposed to be extremely carefully monitored and I hardly think our inconsequential ten minute conversations constituted any sort of monitoring whatsoever. But I began to feel better and better – I loved the new drug.

At the end of April, I was stunned and thrilled with myself, as I had **finally** stood up for myself in the face of my family. I had actually said what I wanted and what my own personal needs were – something I'd rarely done. I knew that perhaps I would become an outcast to much of the family, whom I had always adored. What a huge step. The culmination of this giant leap forward was a long, carefully crafted letter to my sister Lucy with whom I shared a house. Writing it was the hardest thing I've ever done.

I wanted out of the difficult ownership for many reasons and I knew she did not want to sell. My desire to do it was well-founded, I still believe. However, some of my close friends began to think that my 24-hour attention to writing the letter and my pride in it were becoming an obsession and the obsession was getting manic. I think by the end of the month, things were already well under way down hill.

My friend Susan had been privy to all the revisions and tweakings of the letter, but when I insisted on talking about it during an entire lunch with an older friend I hardly knew, she became very concerned. *"Was I the only one thinking this was over the top? I trusted my radar, but what should I do? There's a period of time leading up to an episode when the signs are appearing, behavior is getting more erratic, but it's hard to trust in it. Those close to Pol were being pulled along on the wave, not willing to believe it would grow out of control. Now we know, then we didn't."*

There was a visit with Harriet and her husband in May, when apparently I kept telling her how cheerful I was feeling – enough to send off some alarms in her head. *"The best description of you then was 'brassy' and Don should always be on the look-out for this attitude. You were talking a little louder, moving a little faster in May."* She called from the car as they left the Cape, very concerned, noting that, *"the higher you got, the less sensitive you were to what others thought and felt."*

And Susan again, as the end of May approached: *"At another lunch, we had had to wait a while to be seated, but Pol's agitation and self-proclaimed state of starvation far exceeded the situation. The wait was much more of a problem for her than for anyone else and I watched with discomfort as my friend Polly, a polite, mature, empathetic woman who has waitressed herself, became pushy, demanding and rude. She asked for extra lettuce for a huge salad we hadn't even been served yet, extra dressing to accommodate it, extra lemons twice to have with her water. She continued to eat long after we had finished our lunch.*

"The uncharacteristic narcissism was showing itself, another red flag. It is one of the most prominent manic behaviors, as the normally humble and grounded suddenly become The Funniest, The Most Brilliant, The Always Right, The Only. Polly, usually so concerned with others, became self-centered."

My friend Mykee remembers my uncharacteristically aggressive behavior at the time: *"You insisted on cutting one of my best peonies and I hadn't said you could. Normally you would never do that."*

Other friends, who saw me more often and took their responsibilities as members of my "bipolar team" very seriously, were worried and came to the house to share their unease. *"The problem is you are so much fun to be with and so fiercely bright that most people don't want to see that you're not yourself."* To them and to Harriet I responded, "The therapist thinks I'm doing just fine."

Harriet noted later that the therapist didn't see *"that your happiness was a very real indication of how badly you needed some sort of stabilizer. You do have an air of whimsicality. You're extemporaneous without being compulsive. People couldn't imagine the red flag for what it was."*

I find this therapist completely responsible for what happened to me, although as I have said before and must repeat, in the early stages of mania, we are infinitely clever and manipulative. Perhaps she would have had to spend many hours with me to see my impending breakdown. But, there was no follow-up when Harriet tried to enlist her help as the mania welled up in Maine shortly after our last session together. *"She denied it was happening, would not return phone calls, and when she finally did, called in wrong prescriptions, and so forth."* Though I've tried, it's too hard for me to forgive this person for wreaking such havoc with my life through the new prescription and then lack of attention to its results.

Once in Maine that early June, I couldn't keep track of the wonderful ideas that rushed into my brain and couldn't wait to share them. I was sure that the potential titles for my book would fascinate my friends: "Why Bipolar is a Gift, not a Disease," "Could This be Better Than The Loaves and the Fishes?" And since I found myself so terribly amusing, "How I Became Funnier than the Whole World, including my Sister Harriet – The Jury is Out on Robin Williams."

My friends were again appalled at my racing thoughts, my inability to stop talking and settle down. *"You were in constant motion, going in 100 different directions, spinning your wheels. You were **clearly** in trouble."* I very much wanted reassurance that they thought I was OK and it was totally frustrating when I didn't get it. I spent hours trying to convince them and failed.

Except for the short book titles, my thoughts were coming too fast for me to verbalize coherently. I would begin a sentence with some specific ending in mind, but before I got there, several more thoughts would crowd in and there was no way to keep track of anything I'd meant to say. Any complicated thought was impossible to express unless other people repeatedly questioned me or interrupted to force my attention back to the original point.

An idea I remembered from a newspaper a year or so earlier particularly entranced me and I told my friends about it: "There's a 60-year old woman in Rome who's just had a baby. As soon as the summer's over, I'm going over there, find that doctor and get pregnant. I've known forever that I'd be a great mother and I always planned to have lots of little blond children." Everyone laughed at this, but I was completely serious. It certainly didn't matter what Don wanted – it didn't occur to me to ask or to care.

The same was true with my projected facelift, to be performed by excellent surgeons at a highly reputed, inexpensive hospital in Thailand. Don was especially horrified at this. When subjected to this barrage of ideas, a friend of mine who has spent decades in the field of medicine and medical ethics, told me later that for the first time in his life, he'd thought, *"This person should be on drugs."*

An enormous old inn set perfectly on top of a large field leading down to the ledges and waters of Blue Hill Bay hosts a concert each summer of terrific musicians, ethnic food, craft vendors. A magnificent celebration. We really looked forward to listening to the music, visiting with friends, enjoying the beautiful spot.

In the last week of June, it was clear to everyone that I had gone over the edge again, talking incessantly, engaging strangers, trying to share my overwhelming feelings of joy and the brilliant ideas crowding my brain. The volunteers at the booth for the little day camp I had been scheduled to man let me know politely that, *"Thanks, but we don't need your help after all, we ended up with enough people."* My stepdaughter's extended family, on a visit to Maine, sat awestruck and silent in the face of my lengthy (and of course always cheerful) diatribes. They and everyone else I came across were dumbstruck, as my behavior had again become too frantic and frightening.

"I want to see the manager," I demanded at the front desk of the inn. "He has treated me incredibly rudely and I need to tell him in person. He owes me an apology right away." The man did not appear. To chastise him, I lifted several glasses off the bar, planning to take them home as recompense. My friends tried to dissuade me: *"Don't you care that that would be stealing?"* It seemed perfectly just to me: well-brought up little girls from

Princeton, New Jersey don't brook rudeness easily and especially not when manic. My friends finally took me home, fighting (albeit good-naturedly) all the way.

Right around this time I had another, to me completely wonderful idea: The campfire pit at our house was going to be the absolutely perfect spot for our new restaurant. No need at all to advertise – people were constantly looking for places to eat nearby. Probably the smells would be so good that they were all we'd need to entice people there, no problem. The granite pit had a six or seven foot circumference, a huge grill, a gorgeous view of the pond, Adirondack chairs Don had made, a lovely yard for overflow guests.

We had discussed the idea with a Spanish friend at least 15 years earlier. It involved buying extremely expensive meats, making beautiful salads and sangria. Very simple. Guests arrived, the meats were cooked to a T, the moon was shining. Heaven. My only question was, "Why can't we start today?" I never questioned my ability to pull this one off and of course it would be a big money maker, even though money didn't matter to me any more. I knew everything I touched would turn to gold.

Money has been always been a big problem for me, growing up as the child of parents whose rich families had lost everything in the Depression. Scrimping and saving were the way we grew up, and the idea of taking out a loan was beyond the pale. Somehow the fear of becoming a bag lady had taken hold in me – apparently this is not uncommon for women my age. The difficulty

I've had for decades in spending has been a burden to me and to others close to me. I've been extremely penurious, especially after giving up my pottery business and only having occasional income from mediation.

An example of the hurtful effect of this psychosis occurred over 20 years ago when I refused a collect call from a stepdaughter. "Why couldn't she just call person to person collect so we could get the number and call her back?" I railed at Don. "Doesn't she know how expensive collect calls are? Doesn't she have any idea of how close to the vest we're living?" Old telephone habits from my parents dictated these strict rules, but for her it was unforgivable and I heard about it viciously in 2003.

All that changes when I'm manic. The first time I experienced the joy of spending without anxiety was in 2000. I bought all the tasty little fancy grocery items I'd always denied myself – what fun. I spent hours in one store, positively enthralled by what I could buy now with pleasure. We were lucky in 2005 that all I spent were a few hundred dollars on ten copies of my friend Linda Greenlaw's cookbook, written with her mother. That I paid in advance for the order was most surprising to the saleswoman, who assured me it was unnecessary. "No problem," I replied insouciantly. Don couldn't stop this purchase, but he successfully prevented me from buying a house I'd set my heart on for my nephew in Blue Hill and one for my friend in Newport.

Wild, uncontrolled spending is one of the hallmarks of a full-blown manic experience. Fortunes have been lost due to manic depression. The impact on the patient's family is often the most harmful and long-lasting. In my case, family members urged my husband to separate our finances as completely as he could. In addition, Harriet noted, *"Separating the property and any money was something Don could actually do, as opposed to the helplessness he was feeling."*

Later on, when I was not manic but vastly depressed, the fact that this separation had happened -- they'd all said it **had** to happen -- was devastating for me. We even had to hire another lawyer for Don, instead of the one we had shared for years. How could I have been so terrifying, I wondered again and again. And to top it off, Lucy had removed me from the joint account we shared for the house – another tremendous blow.

The costs of my illness have been in the thousands and thousands of dollars. For instance, because the service for our cellphones was not as promised, I threw them both out in a fit of temper – hundreds of dollars – and then hundreds more when I kept changing the options of the new server. The speeding tickets I incurred as I roared around the countryside in July of 2005 were steep, despite my subsequent efforts to appeal to the police departments of both states. Many medical expenses, like blood tests, ambulances, and most importantly, drugs, are not covered by insurance. For victims of mental illnesses, many of these costs will continue forever.

Not surprisingly, I was furious when I landed again in the hospital. Once again control had been wrested from me and it would be en enormous waste of time in my now valuable life. Somehow Harriet convinced me to sign myself in, but she sat there aghast with the intake psychiatrist as I conversed cogently and totally on track. *"But finally, finally, you launched into a long and inappropriate discourse on puppies."* The psychiatrist recognized immediately I was in the right place. I don't remember a thing about it.

My memory of so much is gone, unless I have notes, and it seems this is true for other victims of this illness. A patient cited by Goodwin and Jamison in the '90's: *"Madness carves its own reality. It goes on and on and finally there are only others' recollections of your behavior – your bizarre, frenetic, aimless behavior – for mania has at least some grace in partially obliterating memories."*

This time I thought I might like my gorgeous Persian psychiatrist – a lovely woman I never saw without her assistant, Debra, her Sancho Panza. For a while it occurred to me that maybe we could actually have some meaningful conversations. No dice. *"Good morning Polly, did you sleep well? How do you feel today? Would you like to discuss anything this morning?"* As usual, it irritated me enormously that this doctor could make any judgments about me, my care, the length of my stay, based on virtually nothing.

The doctor kept me on the medication prescribed in February, Lamictal, as I insisted it made me so happy. Consequently, my ten-day stay at this hospital only served to prolong and increase my mania – the weeks that followed my release were a nightmare for all involved. I've asked my sister and Don why they thought the psychiatrist did not put me back on a calming drug, even if I refused the more traditional bi-polar medications like Lithium or Depakote (I may have). *"You were too strong for her. You were so self-contained and articulate, so credible and manipulative that you convinced them you were all right to be released."*

I was hell-bent on staying on the Lamictal, since I was sure it had turned my life around. Another way I was sure to make my fortune was as the spokesperson and poster child for the drug – a first-hand paean to its magnificent success in changing a quite sad and depleted person into a creative, articulate and charming one – me. The company would have no need for anyone else to advertise the efficacy of the medication, as I would be so good. (It has in fact been successful in many instances, but as I said earlier, it must be carefully monitored and clearly does not work for everyone. No drug does. In my case, it only served to exacerbate my vulnerability to the illness and caused irreparable damage to my life and that of my family.)

No group discussions, air, exercise – it was all exactly the same as in other institutions. "How can anyone imagine that depriving even crazy people of air and exercise is therapeutic?" I wrote in a letter to the head of the unit. "This seems to be only a drug-dispensing facility. And the staff's rudeness and disdain for patients might be excusable if these attitudes weren't present in almost every conversation or order – the whole vocabulary and body language caused in large part by their boundless stupidity." My conclusion was it was caused by "the need of insecure people for power." And further, "I am a professional mediator and would be very happy to help you resolve some of these clear weaknesses in staff/patient relations." Imagine what she must have thought, if she even read the letter!

Emil Kraepelin presents the other side: *"With their surroundings the patients often live in constant feud. They interfere in everything, overstep their rights, make arrangements which they are not entitled to make... They have no understanding whosoever for the unseemliness of their behavior; they do not comprehend at all why everything they do is taken amiss, are astonished in the highest degree at the complications which arise, but get over it with a few jests."*

My passion for reaching out to my friends and family on the telephone was particularly annoying to the staff: *"You've been spending MUCH too much time on the phone ever since you got here. From now on, you can only make a call at the beginning of any hour and you can't talk more than fifteen minutes during that hour."* As it turns out, it would have been best if I'd been cut off completely – I did real emotional damage to friends in these conversations. My rage was explosive and mean when someone suggested, for instance, that one of my ideas didn't make sense, or tried to persuade me to go to sleep. And with no rules, the hurt I inflicted on so many only increased once I was released from the hospital.

I tried to fight back against the staff by listing the various mental disorders on the blackboard in the rec room. Not surprisingly, they were erased two or three times before I gave up. Next, I wrote a note in Spanish about how they were little fishes in a big sea – bad, evil people without power. And finally my last blackboard offering was a list of my favorite books: *"Krakatoa," "King Leopold's Ghost," "Kite Runner," "Winter's Tale," "Time and Again," "Dark Tide," "Don't Let's Go To The Dogs Tonight," "Scribbling the Cat."* I imagine the staff thought this was a fairly banal act so they let the titles stay for a while.

Every single one of my actions must have been very irritating to a group that was just trying to hold a difficult ward together. I babbled away incessantly, ran around starting activities, engaged patients who were happy just looking at a bingo board or year-old magazines. As far as I know, no new medication had been administered to calm me down, so I just got higher and more out of control.

My frenzied flow of ideas continued unabated, however annoyed I would get with the staff, with Don, or with other patients. My best idea (and I still believe it would be very educational and also attract a wide audience) was to produce a television show, a sit-com. We would develop stereotypical characters representing a wide spectrum of mental illnesses and distinct personalities. I made more notes on the patients and their problems with an eye to the show. Through the use of humor and some sort of plot, I would gradually and insidiously inform the great unwashed public about the variations of disorders, show how patients could be and were treated, how families are affected by their loved one's problems, etc. The grand goal would be to show that mentally ill people are just that – ill people – and that they need understanding, compassion and with that an openness to the idea of allowing and possibly aiding their re-entry into the world.

A visit on the Oprah Winfrey Show would also go a long way toward achieving this same goal, I figured, and I enlisted the help of my friend Susan. I called her, apparently very agitated and excited, asking her to get in touch with Oprah about setting up a TV interview about my book. I explained to her this was going to be the definitive book on bi-polar disease, and an incredible success. *"Pol might even have some plastic surgery done first so she could look good on television. If there's one thing Pol is NOT, it's vain."*

Though the sit-com and the Oprah visit still make sense to me, the fact that I wanted to adopt a cat from the newspaper was questionable. Someone wanted to find a new home for a gorgeous Maine coon cat, my favorite kind. I called the family and assured them: "Of course we'll take it. My husband will be over this afternoon." It didn't turn out that way, as Don immediately vetoed the idea. I was beside myself with astonishment and fury. "Don, I hate you right now. You do not have a CLUE what this is like. No power of decision, no air, no home, no Pascal. You won't even understand enough to give me the only thing I want more than my freedom – that cat. Why not??? I promised to give it to someone if you/we didn't want it. Pascal loves cats. Are you worried about freedom of choice – i.e. **you** haven't chosen this cat? The only time you've fought was to deny me the cat. Even forgetting my failed misery, what possible harm could it have been, to babysit someone's cat and then give it away? Why was this an appropriate time to dig in your heels? WHY???"

Anger became my watchword, nothing seemed very funny any more. One of the patients said to me nastily, *"It's not up to you to clean up and organize the kitchen."* Another refused to let me sit at her table, *"You talk too much and I can't stand to be around you."* And the doctor and Sancho Panza seemed the most ridiculous, asking me when I came into the office with a huge grin of happiness, *"And how are you feeling today?"* As if there were any question.

And Don was the devil incarnate in my mind. A proposed chapter heading for one of the books I was planning: "I am so SICK of everyone being sorry for Don." He could do nothing right in my eyes, even though he was driving over an hour each way to the hospital, just to be abused by his witchy wife.   In my notes I ranted and railed against him: "How could you be so insensitive? Why don't you ever listen to me? Where is Pascal – you promised to bring her and now she's not here. Don't you know how it makes me feel when you tell someone I am manic? You said you'd call and you didn't. You said you'd come at 2:00 and you didn't get here til 2:30." Horrible and it only got worse.

My progression towards losing control of my temper would always begin with astonishment and surprise, lead to frustration, end in anger. I made firm resolutions to take deep breaths and walk away but they usually didn't work. Concentrating on keeping my voice low when making a point proved impossible and I'd end up yelling at Don. But note my self-awareness: "So, last clue of mania. Can't not yell or walk away."

It seems that before, during and after this hospitalization, although I was constantly full of self confidence and certainty that I was all right, much better than all right, I knew at the same time that I was indeed manic. An evidence of this is my love affair with book titles, some of which were major cries for help. Take the early ones, for instance: "Just Ask Me If I Think I'm Perfect, Or Just Lock Me Up," or "I Might Have Another Manic Episode, So Please Just Lock Me in a Room," or "Lock Me in a Room: The Perfect Jump Start Toward Treating Bipolar Disorder." I was so pleased with them at the time, but I think these are telling examples of some recognition of my mania and my wish for someone to help me, since I couldn't help myself.

That the psychiatrist released me after ten days was, as a close friend said, *"hideous, a failure, dangerous."* Although Sancho Panza made an appointment for me in a month with another doctor, there was no suggestion of post-hospitalization structure or therapy. The medication which had failed to avert the onset of the episode and allowed it to go out of control was still in place, though the psychiatrist gave me another prescription to be taken with it. (Of course I didn't fill it – I felt too good and knew I didn't need it.) It was clear to Don that the release was completely wrong, but his hands were tied by his wife's clever dealings with the doctor and perhaps also by patients' rights.

As John Custance wrote, *"The horses of passion and*

instinct have run away. All brakes or clogs or checks on the whole functioning of the psycho-physical mechanism are removed; the channels of instinct are freed; the libido can flow where it will." This is how I came out of the hospital.

Chapter Six:

The Beginning of the Aftermath

I'd like to write a poem about
how it was when Pol was going through her – episodes –
that's friendly
It was shit, awful, crappy, a great black pit for me
to wade through
with no way out

"So Don, why are you so sulky and quiet?" I asked him on the way home from the hospital. Why can't you be happy for me that I'm finally free and out in the air? I've told you a million times how horrible it is to be jailed like that." I just couldn't understand and screamed at him angrily and loudly in the car. One of the most difficult and typical problems that mental illness causes in families is the fury the patient directs straight at them. The patient naturally blames the close family for arranging the incarceration and any suggestions that run counter to his plans. The fact that Don, the closest to me, was always the brunt of my fury, is perfectly normal.

Later on, though, on our return home, after I had apparently given him quite a speech about our lives, I did make a note that he probably couldn't hear me because he was so hurt and exhausted and miserable. At least in my self-absorption I could notice that. Being together in the house didn't seem to work, so I sat down in front of the barn to write him a letter.

I loved writing that letter. It made me so happy that I didn't even practice my life-long excessive attention to grammar and spelling. The setting was beautiful, the sun was going down over the gorgeous pond, Pascal was right there. I could calmly explain everything to Don who would then be content and let go of his doubt that we could stay married – a doubt he'd expressed a few times in the last ten days. He was already getting a lot of questions about our marriage and some pressure to get out of it. I knew he would discard that idea once he read my eloquent, apologetic and thoughtful letter.

It was quite a sweet recognition that he had loved me in "my very flawed state," which I went on to describe at length and in extremely self-deprecating terms. I spelled out the most egregious of my mistakes and awful personality faults, ending with, "Why would a nice perfect guy like you love me, since I was so pathetic in my soul?" My emphasis was that in spite of all this negativity, his love had been a constant for 27 years. "That you think we could possibly not be able to be together astounds me but I understand it – My disease took over, it wasn't your fault, you tried and couldn't handle it. No one could."

The letter was my chosen means of fighting for him, laced with what I considered proof of my love and worthiness to stay married. I outlined how thrilling it was to rid myself of the Watcher – the evil that keeps the heart and mind separate. I wrote about anger and how it would never be so ferocious again. That I would repair and improve any old hurts with his daughters – maybe my next book would be: "How I Finally Became a Perfect Stepmother After 27 Years." And on and on. My only request was that we would set up times for him to listen to me. I hoped he'd ask me about the parts of the letter I hadn't made clear.

As I went into the house to give it to him, I was convinced that I'd made a completely convincing case and he would not want to split up after he read this marvelous letter. But though I considered myself only beautifully cheerful and optimistic, Don was trying to cope with the terrible fact that I had been let out of the hospital totally out of control, probably worse than when I went in since the mania had been building for another two weeks. But he hadn't yet given up.

In the throes of a manic episode, as I have described, a victim's thoughts are racing, tremendously facile and grandiose. There is really no need or desire for input from others – he has all the answers and they are better, more intelligent and they come fast and furious. Don writes: *"It became obvious I was the block to the aspirations of far flung grandeur."* His sorrow at the resultant loss of communication of heart and soul is evident in this next poem.

Where's the fairness
in a day I've become
extinct
sidelined to the bench
no more to feed the love
of kindred thoughts
what's sad is
She seems to mean it.

My reasonable intentions to please Don and avoid stress (recommended by the psychiatrist) soon disappeared as I was let loose in the world that early July, 2005. My friends had been relieved about the hospitalization but were immediately appalled when I was released in such terrible shape. Apparently I roamed around the house all night, talking to myself, writing on the computer for hours at a time, talking endlessly on the phone. And listening to very loud music, dancing, laughing. I don't remember a thing about it, so here is Don's recounting of the pattern of those days, and then one specific one.

"Time faded into meaningless episodes of what used to be normal living. I didn't understand it. Mornings became assemblages of plans that crashed upon each other with frenzied rapidity. Lunch might happen. It was the one clinging constant. Although it was fast losing its grip in the rush of larger goals.

"One sailing afternoon Pol became convinced that I had forgotten how to sail. I couldn't gybe. I didn't understand

the new mooring pick-up method downwind with more speed. I'd had a stroke. The doctor in the Emergency Room was perplexed, but Pol knew she was right.

"Evenings blended into unending periods of anticipation. Of worry, of constant sense of strain to outguess the coming time. The noises stop, the car is gone – peace – for a minute – for an hour or two. Do I worry or say the hell with it. It's becoming a mess in the house.

"8:00 p.m. The car returns. Blaring hard rock or Dixie Chicks. Supper – forget it. Better to ride the edges of the sound and the fury. Pick up where I can. Suggest something more reasoned? No. I have learned that's to no avail.

"10:00 p.m. The mattress on the bed feels the same. The house vibrates with music, singing, moving furniture. Thoughts out loud. The cupboards are being re-arranged, or maybe torn down. A wineglass shatters, a plate hits the floor. Laughter. The volume goes up.

"Midnight: Pascal and I cling to our mattress. Maybe the weight of night will hit us with oblivion. Pascal seems lucky but maybe she is faking. I think we both feel (know) that we are lucky in having this one sanctuary.

"1:00 a.m. A cork pops, gurgle sounds, something heavy falls: it's Pol. Sympathy springs forward but loses hold amid the language from downstairs. Crash, scraping of furniture, the kitchen door slams. In the sudden quiet I wonder if I'll recognize the house by daylight.

"3:00 a.m. Quiet rational talking on the phone to North Carolina. Excited but insistent and enthusiastic. I hope

Bets had some sleep early in the evening. The call drones on and this becomes a quiet time of night to doze.

"5:00 a.m. The phone goes silent. The house is tomblike. Do you go and look or drift away to sleep, the better course; as you know it will all be starting again. Confusion and mind-numbing dislocation."

Don's poem written a year later about that night:

3:00 a.m.
the dishes rattle
the phone conversation wanders on
splintered glass reverberates –
lights are on –
the night is so slow –
I wish I could talk to Pascal
I can of course but we
lie like zombies in the darkened room
waiting for
something

My mood careened wildly from jubilant to infuriated, and fighting with Don was constant. He writes: *"At the heights of the 'Eden Express' as someone has called it, I was 'big time' the bad guy. I could do no right. It was becoming an impossible situation. The house reverberated with her banging around, breaking glasses and coffee cups, generally causing havoc. There seemed to be no end to what chaos she could create and I began to worry about the house."*

Rachel told me this old farmhouse
has been here since 1890
I'll bet it has seen life and love
and hate
and life
I wonder if it ever saw destruction
of its soul
its hominess
It has that so strong
it may be tough to lose
no matter how she tries.

I began to put Don's things outdoors, first pictures, then clothes, the books and pieces of furniture. He describes coming over to the house (he'd been at the new house we'd built and had on the market) and finding dozens of books piled on the porch in the rain. He gave up and moved to the other house. Who could blame him?

The windows retch with babel and with clatter
and vomit clothes and books upon the ground –
my friendly green lawn my space
like Baghdad – bespoiled.
But chaos grips the peace and writhing binds its python
grip
it must not know the life it's spewing out –
or why.

My major reaction was surprise that we were truly splitting up, but I was quite happy about it, since I really couldn't bear to be around him. I happily told friends we were going to get a divorce, I was going to be very nice about it and would even help him find another woman. Not surprisingly, he rejected my offer. But from the following note, it seems clear I really couldn't contemplate life without Don.

"My astonishment over my husband (of 27 years)'s inability to cope and lack of interest in learning to live with me in my new 'incarnation' is boundless. He indicated he wished he could go along with me on my journey but his psyche or his energy or his whatever just wouldn't allow it.

"This was the man who devoted almost 30 years to my happiness and lost that interest in continuing – suddenly, surprisingly.

"It took almost two weeks after I was discharged from my third incarceration before I realized he had given up, thrown in the towel. On the phone, he was as usual – kind, caring, thoughtful.

"In person he was the devil incarnate. There was no good idea I could have – even to suggest he might like to go sailing on this wonderful boat we'd been longing to be invited on – all was negative, put down, dismissed usually rudely, every once in a while I'd be told he'd think about it.

"So I could make no suggestions nor do anything right in his eyes – nothing. And this went on until we were separated and I realized my vision of life was now unacceptable – our marriage was irrevocably over. It had been so nasty that good riddance was/is my only thought..

"A few vestiges of the demon were still around, like the morning he kicked me out of his new house. Now I think he has just passed on and isn't very interested in engaging with me in any way – who knows.

"I've felt quite secure that we'd still do things together – go to Paris, go skiing, sail – but now am not sure as he has almost, at least temporarily, disengaged. This may change as our lives still can enrich each other's, specifically creatively – the raku, the stone garden, maybe that's it – jesus.

"So what happens now? Was he so deeply hurt by my craziness or is it really the new independence and self esteem that have taken over my soul?"

So there I was, living alone, totally involved with painting the house, talking constantly on the phone to friends, having better and better ideas every moment: discussions about manic depression at the Community Center, a kids' book in Spanish, volunteering anywhere in the world in a school. My ideas and realizations made me "choke or laugh out loud or just be awestruck. All my major negative personality deficiencies started to erode." And a vow: "Now I still have many of them but they will be (a) more controlled and (b) I'm working on them, like ANGER." I was completely self-confident and self-righteous.

Chapter Seven:

Road Trips

Whoa!
I seem to be falling
Through the one hole in my life
I never saw
Where is the bottom?

Though I was completely enthralled with my house painting project, there seemed to be even better, more enticing reasons to abandon it and rush all over the eastern seaboard -- one of which was to buy a Prius. What was so strange about wanting a Prius badly enough to drive from northeastern Maine to southwestern New Hampshire to find one? Who cared how far away the Sales Office was? I drove off excitedly. That it was after business hours and I could never get to the closest one in

New Hampshire that day didn't bother me a bit. I had all the money in the world to stay in a motel.

That the salesman whom I met the next morning should be concerned that I didn't have my license or a credit card was ridiculous – what did it matter? I told him I had wonderful credit so why was there any question? Well then, could I use the phone and get my husband to bring me the appropriate documents? Although Don refused, I persisted. Time went on. I knew I would drive off in my new car.

When the sales manager ultimately (and furiously) kicked me out of this New Hampshire dealership, I was amazed. How silly of him to lose that sale and his commission. Poor ignorant fellow. Wait til he got home and admitted his mistake to his wife. Who knows where I drove after that – very carefully and fast. My preoccupation with purchasing a Prius remained paramount throughout those ever-wilder weeks, and a year or so later, I did get one.

There was something about driving – at least when I was driving, no one was trying to give me advice, to tell me to calm down, to control me. My friend Grace said, *"You were really quite amenable to everything I suggested except not getting in the car and zooming off."* Efforts to get me out of the car, to get medical attention, to get some sleep were in vain. Friends and family were positive I would kill myself on the road – I, on the other hand, was very proud of my safe driving.

Who cared anyway that on the way to Cape Cod I'd gotten lost and driven literally hundreds of miles out of my way? I was just having such fun, talking for hours on the cell phone, making some tapes, thinking important thoughts. Limericks especially kept floating into my head, amusing me inordinately, and of course innumerable book titles. And then there was music – loud, loud Cd's – Dixie Chicks, Ian and Sylvia, Fleetwood Mac, Peter Frampton. I must have listened to the Dixie Chicks' "Top of the World" hundreds and hundreds of times. I was so proud they had stood up and spoken against the President.

(After this episode was all over, it took ten months for me to be able to listen to music again. I was terrified that listening to music in the car would bring my mania back. The dial was perpetually set on NPR and I would panic if someone had changed the channel and music came on. I can still see exactly where on a small road near our house in Maine, in early June of 2006, I slipped in an Abba tape of my sister's. Touching the volume control took a huge act of will, but gradually I dared to do it and it was all right. And I continued along my way, singing first tentatively and then more loudly to the familiar tunes. What a triumph and renewal of joy.)

Not surprisingly, Don wasn't having any fun at all after I took off for the Cape. He'd found a note I'd written as I excitedly left on the trip, saying basically that I'd rather not die on the road, but if I did, it would be perfectly all right with me, since I was finally so happy now. I had conquered death! Drums rolled, people were stationed at bridges and ferries, police departments were alerted. Actually, it would have been great if I'd had a minor accident. No such luck.

Harriet knew I was headed to the Cape and called Mykee and Marcia, asking them to meet her and her husband John to head me off at the Bourne Bridge and convince me to enter a hospital. Marcia describes their errand of mercy as *"either a wild goose chase, a helpful mission, or a Thelma and Louise drive. We met Hat and John and stood around talking about the futility of what we were doing, swore to uphold each other through any other feeble or successful attempts to capture the elusive, light speed traveler that was our cherished friend."* Who knows where I was that night – I was not to be found.

(Again though, at my wildest, I somehow had an inkling that I was over the edge. I never would have admitted it to anyone. In one of my tapes I mentioned the beauty of the paintings of Maine artist Tom Curry and reminded myself that though I was crazy now and adored his work, I should check it out when I wasn't crazy and see how I felt about it. Those little glimmers.)

Eventually I did make it over the bridge, having driven multiple hours out of my way, and getting lost in Cambridge, my college town, for hours. I felt the Harvard police treated me harshly as I circled and circled the same blocks, ending up in some very dark and dingy streets far away from the Square. Susan had been prepared for me to spend the night.

"I had the guest bed made, her favorite food, a bedside book. She never showed. At 7:00 AM. the next morning, I got a call from Pol that she was 'somewhere' in my neighborhood, but couldn't find my house. I asked for a street name; she drove around until she could read one. She was, indeed,

right around the corner. I gave her the directions, she didn't show. Another call came in – she was farther away. Finally, I asked her to just pull over and I drove to where she was, to lead her home. I could see her frustration, yet in true manic fashion, it was the fault of the street signs and the road planners, and certainly no cause for concern. She had apparently driven all night, but where was unclear – the trip should have taken six hours."

I was looking forward to having lunch with friends, all of whom, unbeknownst to me, were primed to outline my behavior to me and steer me toward the hospital. Susan wrote later that: *"I had trouble with the deceit aspect, but we were all very concerned by this point. To force someone into treatment, they must be a threat to themselves or to others. We felt the threat might lie in crazy driving or poor choices. Pol arrived wearing no shoes, and though initially happy to see the assembly of friends, she became defensive as soon as Marcia began to talk, expressing her concern."*

Marcia picks up the story: *"As we were studying the menu, the men in blue arrived. Don and Hat had spoken with the police in Eastham. They asked Polly to come outside where they had blocked her car and interviewed her as to her safety, her driving, her plans and her destinations."*

Susan describes how *"the cop was trying to establish her sanity by asking questions like 'Who is the President of the United States?"* Pol is an extremely intelligent person, and this all struck her as ridiculous and also confusing. *"Why are they asking me all these stupid questions?"* It struck me then how hard it is for others to respect the dignity of a person in the throes of mania, because their behavior is so *outlandish. And they are so sure they are right, fine, great, in control. But they are not in control of their actions; they are suffering from an illness and deserve to be treated with care and respect..*

"This may take a huge amount of patience and may not even be well-received by the patient. But just as you would not be angry at a sick child for vomiting or an elderly person for bed-wetting, despite the hassles involved, so should you not blame the mentally ill for their behavior, even when it's almost intolerable. They are not in control, or even aware, of what they say and do."

Marcia takes it up again: *"With considerable skill and intelligence she deferred and deflected all queries and returned to lunch, furious with her family who had sent the police. "Pol,' said her friend from paddle tennis, 'I believe you trust me and know I wish you no harm. I want you to understand that you are not safe now and you must get help.'*

"Polly rose from the table, went to her car, and drove away in fury. We were left with no appetites, an angry restaurant owner who wanted relief from this drama, and some patrons. We ordered lunch and ate it, sharing our guilt, our inadequacy, our emptiness, our hurt, and our despair."

And Susan writes, *"We had no idea where she would go. We had failed. I now wonder how we thought we could succeed. She was already there, in the irrational state of mania. She was already the self-proclaimed queen of the universe. We were too late. We had driven her into exile."*

Somehow I drove safely back to Maine, assuredly

listening to my loud music and having outrageously interesting thoughts. I can't remember a thing about it, but soon thereafter, Don and I set off together to the wedding of the daughter of some of our favorite friends. I was very irritable, horribly rude to Don and smoking so much on the trip that he got out of the car half way and took the bus home. Not only had he reached his breaking point, he was convinced his presence only made my mania worse.

It's really due to my cell phone communication with Susan that I know anything about that trip. She came on board when I'd taken a right instead of a left at the lower edge of Lake Champlain and again driven hundreds of miles out of my way, heading north instead of west. She reports: *"There were speeding tickets, more than one. She continued talking to me as she was pulled over one time, simultaneously chatting with the officer and with me. What must he have thought? Not too much, apparently, since he wrote the ticket and sent her on her way."*

Susan reports my lack of success in trading my old car in for a Prius: *"Either there were none on the lot, or she had no money, or it was closing time, or the scenario was far wackier than any of these. I heard from her again from the parking lot of her motel – she had made it at last. It was about 11:30 PM and she was sharing some red wine and a cigarette (Pol doesn't smoke) with a male guest she had just met in the lot.*

"I didn't hear from her until the next afternoon. She'd set off to get her hair hi-lighted for the wedding. A trip to the beauty parlor for her is a unique notion – she has great,

thick hair but doesn't spend any time on it at all. She got lost returning from the appointment, wandering the back roads for hours, almost missing the wedding entirely."

My next misdeed was to alarm the cousins with whom I stayed as I detailed well into the night the miracle of my new happiness, how extraordinary my life had become. I can only imagine how appalled they were at my behavior but as usual, I considered myself at my most charming and interesting. Worse, I angered the grandmother, who made it clear I wasn't welcome in the house during lunch – I went in anyway to collect my bag. And then I got lost on an early morning walk, infuriating my friend, the most darling, clever and cheerful person I know. He and his wife remember kicking me off the island, but I remember deciding it was best for me to leave a day early, since even in my state I could tell my presence was very irritating. *"After all,"* as Susan says, *"They didn't invite this person; they had invited Polly."*

Of all the guilt and shame that I have piled on myself over the course of these manic episodes, this experience was the worst. To have disrupted this beautiful occasion of people so dear to me caused me inordinate pain. I was too ashamed to get in touch with my friends for a year, when I finally got up my courage and called them. It seems no apology had been needed, but of course I hadn't known that. *"We knew the whole thing was beyond your control."* In fact, they had had feelings of guilt for kicking me off the island and that, in combination with what was going on in their lives, had kept them from getting in touch with me.

Susan points out, *"This relationship has been repaired, but as with some repairs, the end result isn't quite the same as the original. Some water under the bridge changes direction on the other side."* I choose to be more optimistic.

Somehow I got back to Maine, but not without a questionable visit to the Baseball Museum in Cooperstown, New York. Why this stands out in my extremely flawed memory is inexplicable. "Where have you placed the portrait of my namesake Mahala Lounsbury, wife of the former Governor?" I asked the director. "No one can find it in the galleries? Not in the computers? Oh please look again," I said politely, I think, but insistently. "I've waited all my life to see it here." I'm pretty sure I finally just gave up. And as far as I know, I didn't get lost returning to Brooksville and Don.

Chapter Eight:

It All Falls Down

At some point at the end of July, my wild road trips and outrageous behavior came to an end in Newport, where my close friend Meg lives. She and her daughters had visited me in the hospital a month earlier, and she'd been in constant touch with me and with Harriet ever since. The two of them were the only ones I hadn't yelled at, hung up on, chastised on the phone. After we'd been chatting for a while on her front porch, enjoying the sight of First Beach in Newport, some very nice policemen arrived and talked with us in a friendly, non-threatening way.

Apparently the Cape detective with whom Harriet had been working had convinced the Newport police that I was a danger to myself, giving them the license to pick me up. Eventually another police car arrived and they made it clear I had no choice but to go with them to the hospital. Off we went.

I can remember sitting there in a skimpy hospital gown from midnight to dawn, waiting interminably for what I was sure would be my release. My sister Lucy appeared – she and Meg waited it out for hours until the psychiatric hospital in Providence gave the go-ahead for my transfer. We set off for a most awful ride. The back bucket seat of the police car was made of the hardest plastic I've ever felt – the trip was painful and long.

"The worst day of my life bar none. The three most important women, friends, family (Harriet, Lucy and Meg) have caused my incarceration – a jailing with no perceptible limit – up to 10 days. I've almost always thought that I would stay out of jail." It's odd now to re-read those notes and to realize how completely amazed I was that I'd been put away. "Never ever have I imagined such an occurrence," I wrote, seemingly most concerned that without a computer I'd have to do the book draft longhand. "The reality now has surpassed the whole Don chapter. I've even forgotten right now how it goes, I am so blown away by this personal tragedy."

But of course the surprise turned to anger. "Being under others' control is the WORST. Fear of being powerless is sort of like fear on a boat of the wind and the sea. Again imprisoned, at the mercy of either external forces or personal, random forces."

The following note from those first hours in the hospital surprises me, given the many weeks in which I had been so supremely confident of my every move.

"Here I am sailing along so fine seemingly and I am now allowing the thought to penetrate that I am not myself – won't go so far as to say therefore I need to be here. Harriet and Meg have both been crying out for the return of the sensitive Pol – missing in action. I have thought I was there in spades. Don says I'm just not quite there. So what is the difference and where is the shaded perception? I seem so clear to myself, so efficient, neat – where is the edge I am missing?"

Later that day, my sisters, John, Meg and I gathered in an office with my South African psychiatrist, a no-nonsense, thoughtful doctor whom I liked. Don did not come down from Maine. *"At some point,"* he writes, *"I felt that I was an aggravation to Polly's condition more than I could be of help. Better to let a sister or a friend wield the influence."* The doctor asked each person to describe me in detail, in my presence. He heard about their extreme difficulty in obtaining medical attention for me in the past.

Many professionals have written about the nightmare caused by the present inability of families and caregivers to hospitalize a person against his will in a psychiatric facility, *"even when the person is floridly psychotic,"* as Christina Adamec writes. *"In most states, mentally ill people must be a danger to themselves or others before involuntary hospitalization becomes an option, and what that means varies from state to state and even from judge to judge. Why? The civil rights lawyers, again."*

"We need to find ways that optimally balance the rights of both individuals and families," as David Karp says, to

relieve the intolerable strain inflicted by mental illness. And Adamec gets a little more specific: *"A competent and ethical physician or group of physicians would commit a patient for a short-term stay in a hospital. But today it is invariably a judge who decides when a person should be involuntarily hospitalized or ordered to take medication as an outpatient."*

Imagine how disruptive and painful these difficulties were for my immediate family, especially Harriet and Don, who had been very involved in all my manic episodes. This last time and the three weeks that followed my completely useless and dangerous hospital stay (after which there was no scheduled follow-up, no change of medication), clearly had the most impact on them, and of course on me. Throughout my illness, Lucy was constantly forced to revisit the horrors of her own mania and depression in the '60's. All of them must have been so relieved **finally** to find me in the care of a very intelligent, caring professional.

Patty Duke describes the pain of families: *"But no matter what the form or severity of the symptoms, the families of those who are manic-depressive suffer emotions as intense and racking as those experienced by the victims of the disease. They leapfrog from empathy to exasperation, from anxiety to anger, from fear to frustration. They try to be patient and fail. They try to understand, then feel guilty because they can't. Sometimes they make it – the marriage stays intact; the children stay connected; the parents offer support. Sometimes they don't. Friends wear out. Spouses lose patience. Children feel overwhelmed and back off. And the victim of manic depression ends up isolated and alone.*

Whatever the scenario, for every person who is manic-depressive, there are multiple others in agony."

And indeed my family had been in agony, especially Don who saw me every day and towards whom my resentment was most often directed. When mania has produced such an internal hurricane, it becomes terribly important for the victim to hang on to any personal control. His family especially seems to want to remove it. Full of self confidence and power as he is, he has even less desire to be advised, much less controlled, by them. And he's wary of them, as they have probably been involved in past incarcerations – it's all horribly difficult and painful.

The doctor checked out with my family a few facts I'd given him. *"Is it true that she worked for Robert Kennedy for two years? Did she really go walking with Albert Einstein in Princeton? Does she really speak several languages? Was it a fantasy or did she drive a motorcycle across North Africa for ten weeks?"* My family answered that these were not hallucinations – I'd had a pretty interesting life. I was to be medicated according to his prescription: Lithium in combination with the Lamictal, plus a strong anti-psychotic. I was to be kept in the hospital indefinitely. He was firm and held his ground.

Some of his notes indicate that my insight and judgment were very limited, which necessitated an emergency certification. My affect was *"labile"* (unstable). The number of plans I described to the doctor were *"significant for a level of grandiosity and expansiveness."* The word "grandiosity" is used constantly regarding the racing, crazily changing thoughts of a manic episode. It always annoyed me to hear my fabulous ideas described as "grandiose." As always the question of "suicidality" was probed — I never in any episode have had suicidal thoughts.

This facility was a cut above the others by far. Even the way the ward was laid out made much more sense — the staff could observe the patients at all times in the main area and the bedrooms were all around it. There was a smaller room with a television, used for the workshops and group conversations often held several times a day. The staff was distant but polite, walks and cigarette breaks took place predictably at set hours twice a day. Quite a difference from the other institutions I'd been in. My real problem was just passing all those hours a day.

I wrote furiously about betrayal in the first day or so. "You have stolen a huge chunk of my life and part of me hates each of you a great deal. You will never control me again." "I would have done ANYTHING you three (Meg, Harriet, Lucy) had asked – seen (two former doctors), get interim prescription. If you all were still so worried why didn't you TELL ME. Why not a therapist? Why police?"

"But why did those three arrest me? There had to be another recourse, they would have known I'd end up in jail." "The big question, WHY? Were they scared I didn't fit in their little niches?" "Harriet knew best of all about my fear of being imprisoned – how could she do this to me?"

The drugs began to do their work and I became very

sad. I grieved for my feet, for some reason. I was being deprived of my fun, my beautiful life, my painting and fixing the house. "It's irretrievable and I'm inconsolable." Soon all writing stopped, my system slowed down completely. The doctor noted that my improvement was quite dramatic, *"with the patient acknowledging the seriousness of her illness."* Eight days went by til my release and Harriet and I drove in tandem to Martha's Vineyard, where we'd been brought up and still had a home.

At some point during the two or three days I stayed with her, Harriet recalls a time when she, John and I were picnicking on the beach. They were completely flabbergasted to realize that I had *"no clue"* about how I had acted, though *"she knew she'd thrown her husband out of the house after deeply humiliating him for weeks, she couldn't remember anything she'd said to her friends in Maine, so she had no idea how she'd be received and who was saying what."* They finally understood that my fragility and defenselessness were boundless, and the full import of what might actually happen to me in this state struck home. *"Pol was overcome with guilt and confusion, and although she appeared warm and composed, she could not hold up her end of a conversation and was very quiet."*

She continues, *"My husband and I had to find a way (a) to defend her as a person and support her without hesitation but also (b) to warn her that she had said and done some mighty painful things to people she loved. And there would be people who would not forgive and forget. We tried to give her the courage to meet them head-on to explain her illness, but she did know there were many who would not give her the chance."*

And who knew at this time what would happen with Don? Was he going to be able to forgive and forget after all the awful things I'd done to him? The pressure from his side of the family to separate from me was emphatic. If this happened, it would fall to Harriet and John and their kids to take on the responsibility for me. The reality was, in the middle of August of 2005, no one really knew what would happen. Harriet put it best, though, *"Don was toasted by you."*

Chapter Nine:

A Sampling of the Verdict from Friends

I have never seen a person undergoing severe manic episodes such as mine, so it is virtually impossible for me to imagine how frightening I often was. Strangers were afraid and horrified, but my friends for the most part were worried for me – especially that I would kill myself in the car during those three weeks of out-of-control living and road trips.

One old "friend" was, however, afraid that I would come burn down her house, and upon seeing me in the library, her husband told me, *"she rushed home and locked all the doors."* One day after I had become stable again, we saw each other on the dock and she said, *"No, we can't be friends any more. A member of my son in law's family and some other friends have been murdered by people with a mental illness."* (Violence to others is almost invariably caused by not taking medication and the likelihood of a manic depressive harming anyone besides himself is remote.)

Though our friendship had deteriorated in the past years and had therefore lost a great deal of its importance to me, such a summary rejection caught me completely off guard. Don and others assured me that *"the fact that she could not deal with the illness is her problem, not yours."*

I summoned up my courage to call her two years later, to see if she would speak with me during the writing of this book and outline her feelings and reactions to my illness. She refused. *"I've had personal experiences with death due to mental disorders, and I have set up my own boundaries to shield myself."* The fact that I intended this manuscript to be an educational tool designed for people to better understand mental illness (such as that which had affected her) did not dissuade her.

Her feeling that the deep and long-term friendship between our husbands has not been marred by her inability to deal with me is quite surprising, as this has categorically not been true. Their relationship has changed a great deal. The ripples of manic depression touch everyone in unimaginable ways.

As I became aware of the many people, close and more distant friends, whom I had disturbed, sworn at, harassed during my illness, I have apologized and explained. I have asked them if they felt they needed an apology to re-bind our friendship. My sister Harriet, who has been there with me during all these episodes, said, *"an apology would be an insult, it's just a superficial word and concept. I've just been very glad to be able to be there and make a difference."* And everyone else I have queried about this, with the exception of my other sister Lucy, has answered in the negative – that they knew I was in the throes of something beyond my control.

Unfortunately, as I have forgotten so many hours and days and weeks of mania, I did not remember Lucy's part in the trials of those times, of my yelling at her over the phone, of hanging up on her. I was unaware of how closely she was tracking my progress through Harriet. Until ten months after the last hospitalization, I did not know she had been waiting for an apology. I should have guessed. Perhaps I can attribute it to the depression following the last episode, but given our loving 6-decade long relationship, my insensitivity still seems unforgivable.

Just as her need for an apology went unfulfilled for much too long, my need for an explanation from another friend has gone on much longer. Some years ago, I must have said something horrible to her during an episode, as she has been quick to avoid me and will not offer any reason for this. I can't even guess what happened. For those of us who cannot remember so much of what's transpired when we've lost our judgment and control, this refusal to engage and explain is truly the cruelest reaction of all.

Conversations are obliterated from the mind of a victim of mania and even the memory of seeing another person at all disappears. How can one apologize without a clue about what's happened or **even that something**

happened at all? It hurts so horribly and I pray that those who have rejected manic depressives without a reason would consider this a plea at least to bring up their feelings and fears.

After many, many months of horrible examples of how awful it was to be around me or speak with me on the phone, I can readily understand why a friendship would founder and even end. But not being given the opportunity to apologize is the worst.

Another reaction from good friends was a decision not to deal with me any more. Before we'd gone to Maine, they had picked up some red flags that others had not – my overwhelming happiness, my total focus on myself (unlike me and especially odd since one of them was undergoing radiation and I didn't seem to care much), my constant and ultimately boring references to the letter to my sister. Eventually they decided that, *"Allowing you to talk to us endlessly about whatever it was seemed as if it was just enabling you."*

The two decided to cut me off until I shaped up. However, a person in my advanced state of mania does not have the capacity to shape up, and an admonishment to *"take charge of yourself"* does no good. As Mondimore says, *"Telling a manic person to 'slow down and get hold of yourself' is simply wishful thinking: that person is like a tractor trailer careening down a mountain highway with no brakes."*

This reaction only served to irritate me enormously while I was still manic, and I found, upon my dejected return to Cape Cod in the fall, that the nature of our friendships had deteriorated and changed. I knew we needed to talk about it, but I was too shy and demoralized for over a year to bring it up. There was always an awkwardness in our conversations and it was clear to me that our close friendship had become forced.

When I finally suggested a meeting, I discovered that the year before, in the absence of one of these friends, I had spoken several times with her sister who'd been visiting on the Cape that summer. Apparently I had betrayed an important confidence and she, the sister, was shaken enough to refuse to answer the phone again in case I were on the other end. More than three years later, our friendship is still shaky.

My other friend had been involved with me in other manic episodes, trying her best to help. This time, however, she had her own physical challenges in addition to trying to improve or at least maintain her husband's parlous health. His stress during the phone calls from me in my manic state was apparently so extreme that in fact it might have been fatal. Until hearing this, I had thought I'd heard the worst outcomes of my actions – not so.

Both of these people felt that in their decision to cut off our relationship until I had calmed down, they had acted responsibly and as loving friends. When I asked them if they will always be wary of me, they replied yes, but their anxiety would lessen as the years go by. Knowing that I am in a therapist's and a psycho-pharmacologist's care and that I have set up all possible legal methods to put me with a professional before the mania sets in will help them. It's still very sad and I am not optimistic about the return of our mutual trust.

My friend Tim chose a different route and told me he didn't have the time nor the physical health to have me visit when I was manic. I accepted this with equanimity and understanding, since during those July days I was constantly cheerful, with the exception of when I was angry with Don. Tim and I had always been very close and I had no reason to doubt his decision. I learned much later that he did this to protect himself, with the knowledge that there was nothing he could do for me now in my uncontrolled energy and mania.

Though Tim had been in the company of many manic depressives and people taking psychedelic drugs over the years and felt he understood how to get along with people *"in mental extremis,"* he told me he had never seen anyone that completely gone as I was *"because they usually are hospitalized or have done something terrible to themselves – they have disappeared."*

He had realized right away that *"I could not spend more than ten minutes max in your company, even on the telephone – it utterly exhausted me. I just didn't have the strength to get up to that speed. I think it was the first time in these 14 years that I've known you where I just had to deny you, that I just had to say, 'Polly, I cannot do this, goodbye, I cannot be around this energy now.'*

"I think that was my first experience of not only denying you as a friend and saying, 'I can't be your friend under the circumstances – I'll be your friend but we can't talk about it,' but it was also the first time where I just felt this person is too

mad, I can't handle it. It was sort of a humbling experience – well, I'm not Superman."

I asked him if he felt guilty in denying me – his answer was an emphatic no. *"I felt worried about you and wished that I could ease your suffering but at that point you were in a phase of mania where, 'This is the real me, this is how I should be, full of energy, full of ideas, my mind is going like a firecracker, and everything in the whole world is popping out of its sockets and beautiful and everything sounds great and this is the real me.' And in a sense yes it is, when people are like that, but in another sense no, because you cannot sustain it, there is too much energy to sustain itself. It's going to explode or it's going to implode or run out."*

Tim had been around me five years earlier, when the mania had not completely taken over. He remembered well when I came into his home and *"We had a Dire Straits CD playing upstairs in the library, playing quite loud, and you came in and I could just see the energy of that music grab you and fill your body. You got very, very energized by it and said, 'oh yeah, that's what I sound like in so many words,' and you went upstairs to get closer to the speakers."*

Tim was also able to articulate the compassion he felt for me in 2005. *"I worried about the tumble when it came, falling off that high horse, but I also worried about what you were going to do to your social relations as this was the third time. I knew a little bit about the difficulties you had had socially, so I really worried you were going to lose friends, be isolated, have to face a bitter depression and be completely alienated from your friends and the world. And I felt a kind of sorrow over that."*

101

Luckily for me, most of our friends just accepted my odd behavior as an illness and have assured me that though they would be watchful and perhaps more sensitive, they would not be wary of me in the future. Many wished they had been more pro-active. My friend Anne said furiously, *"We should have been much stronger, much clearer, we should have grabbed on by the collar and said 'look, we're going, we're taking you.' I kept thinking, if this were me and we were letting me out, interacting with people in this state, I could never forgive you."*

Throughout the last episode and beyond, our friends were just devastated for Don, whose hands were tied and he had to cope with me every day. As he told a close friend, *"It's just like living in a war zone. I just want to crawl in a hole and go to Spain."* Everyone wanted to help but until the Eastham police finally convinced the Newport police to take me in, there was nothing to be done. My friend Deb was told by a psychiatrist, *"You can't do anything. She needs to be in a hospital, but if she isn't, she'll wear herself out somehow."*

Susan wrote a piece in which she describes what she saw as her responsibility as a friend. *"My role was not to judge or even to counsel. I think it was, ultimately, to hang in there and not to lose sight of the person I knew her to be. I forgave her behavior, I never took it personally. She was never mean or hateful to me, but she surely was with many people she loved. The true ones hung in there, and are still around. Do people change? My belief is they do not. So the friends who did not hang in there, who judged and counseled, are no longer friends. But they never truly were.*

"I trusted she would find her way back and I would be waiting there. Not as though nothing had happened but with exactly the same love I had always had for Pol, not a different person, just a returned one who had been away."

Chapter Ten:

Depression: A Room in Hell with your Name on the Door

Do not be fooled by the relative brevity of this account of my battle with depression. The flip side of the illness of manic depression lasted much, much longer than my periods of mania. Only the very beginnings of a lift in the clouds occurred ten months after my hospitalization in 2005 and later in this chapter I have excerpted a note I wrote more than a year later, still caught in a veil of sadness and despair. In fact it was not until June of 2007 that I consciously began to feel happy, albeit with the help of an anti-depressant.

Depression did not set in immediately after my release from the hospital in Providence in early August of 2005, though I was very unclear and nervous about what was happening between Don and me. He was living in the other house and behaving very carefully and politely toward me. "Where am I going to live?" I wondered. "Can Don and I stay married after all the awful things I've said to him and what he's had to go through?" Harriet and John came to visit around this time and we all had dinner together on pillows in front of the fire in the new house – Don didn't have much furniture yet. The awkwardness of the evening will always stay with me. The presence of one of his daughters, who tried hard to pretend everything was normal, was immensely confusing. When Don asked for her help in purchasing bushes to fill in the empty landscaping in front of the house, I was devastated and didn't know how to express my horror that I'd been replaced.

However, I was determined to begin my intended book describing and detailing my own experience with manic depression. After all, I had been talking about it for years, had several outlines, chapter headings, and so on. I began my research in local libraries, devouring the parts about mania but skipping over those on depression – I just didn't feel my growing confusion as such. The goal for writing was there, but I hadn't wanted to bother with the other side of the illness. I had grown accustomed to the low-level depression my friend had discovered in me in 1994.

Given how my self-confidence was about to hit rock bottom, it's very surprising to me that during these few weeks out of the hospital I was secure enough in myself and my writing to prepare a six-page proposal for the book, sending it to both a close friend in publishing and to the agent of another friend. In fact, I wrote in my notes that I was "optimistic I would develop a new independence of spirit." The optimism was soon to dissipate and then it was gone.

Anxiety was the first clue – I didn't identify it as depression. I just began to be afraid of everything and to feel very timid about Don. Though I had never wanted to live anywhere other than our old farmhouse, I desperately wanted him to invite me to live with him. Here is a note I wrote him in the middle of August:

"Don, I know I've given you a rotten time, but it's over forever. I know you want financial independence, and you'll get it. I won't push you (as long as I can avoid it). I won't force you into any social activities in the winter.

"But ultimately I want us to continue the commitment we made to each other 27 years ago. We can rent or sell this house and you can have as much privacy and space as you require. I understand your devotion to the other house and your pride in it." (He had designed it and been very involved in the building of it.) "I just want us to stay together and respect our independence. Let's not live separately."

My confusion and anxiety worsened as days passed. At some point, Don bought a small boat to replace Aquilon, our old sloop. Though he had no idea if he could even remain married to me, he knew it was a size I could cope with and something we could do together.

Though I was pleased Don had bought it, my terror at the prospect of being on the boat was indescribable.

Despite 50 years sailing and teaching sailing experience in small boats, I was frightened to be asked to do virtually anything – pull in a sail, tie the dinghy to the mooring line. I would double and triple the knots in my panic – the simplest, easiest actions in the world. I only dared to steer because I didn't want to alarm Don, but it was with great trepidation – I was positive I'd run the boat into a ledge or capsize.

Every aspect of life was becoming terrifying to me – seeing people and trying to hold a conversation with them grew more and more difficult. All I wanted was for Don to love me and show it. And at this time, that was impossible for him. It didn't help that I had become tongue-tied and tremendously uncoordinated.

Suddenly I couldn't play tennis, something I'd done perfectly well since about age seven. My brain knew where to stand, how to hit forehands, backhands and serves, but my body had forgotten. My brother in law, John, who had played with me over the years, kindly tried to remind me about basic footwork and proper strokes until mercifully our hour came to an end.

(Later that fall, when I returned to the Cape, the same thing happened with platform tennis. My hope had been that since the court was so much smaller, I'd be able to do it. No such luck. This time the consequences were much worse, as over five years I'd developed a cadre of friends through this game – we'd all improved and brought up our games together. It had become a source of pride, of friendships, a great winter exercise – a pleasure all around.

It is impossible to describe how ineffective I was out there on the court. Neither I nor anyone else could understand what was happening. My athleticism is something, like my decent brain, that I've always taken for granted. Suddenly, the wonderful sport we loved became nothing but torture and humiliation. No words or reminders about how to play did any more good than John's failed attempts to help my tennis. I knew they were right but my body just wouldn't respond.

The words and actions of a person at the height of a manic episode are horrifying to acquaintances and friends, but depression is very, very difficult for them too. The group knew me as a good-humored, talkative, quite athletic person with whom it was fun to play. Suddenly they were faced with a gloomy, ashamed woman with no sense of humor, who apologized the whole time for admittedly terrible performance, and who often burst into tears for no apparent reason.

Susan wrote that she *"really felt Pol should just give it up for a while. It was not a positive experience at all, it was not helping her heal. I often advised my teary friend to give it a break, to stop beating herself up, but there were too many voices encouraging her to stick it out, telling her she'd get better if she kept trying. It was not something she could overcome by will or effort. It lasted til a med revision – she was taking way too much of the wrong thing."*

Harriet told me later, *"You never should have put yourself in this position from the outset, once you knew that playing paddle was impossible for you. When you constantly claim something is your fault, you apologize so profusely, you weaken other people's conception of you. First of all it's not true, and secondly, it reflects your own insecurity, which other people don't have to know about, either. 'Oh my fault, my guilt.' It wasn't fair to them, since they had to spend all their time reassuring you."* Several years later, I'm sure they've not forgotten.)

After mournfully but successfully surviving a trip to the Cape for a wedding and a meeting, I returned to Maine and received an invitation from Don to come live in the house with him. I accepted with alacrity – anything Don wanted to do, I would do. I had virtually no ideas of my own. I agreed with everything he said, pussyfooted around him week after week. Thus began my life as a lapdog.

I can't even imagine how I spent my time. A nasty thing depression does is to remove your ability to read, to focus, to concentrate, to follow a train of thought. So I wasn't reading, I was scared of people, I couldn't sail by myself and could only pretend to enjoy it with Don. I was embarrassed to play tennis since I couldn't hit the ball any more. I'm sure I couldn't bear to go food shopping – my phobia about spending money was back in force. So what was I doing, I wonder? Just getting deeper and deeper into the morass.

In her very special book, *Undercurrents*, Martha Manning writes, *""Depression is such a cruel punishment. There are no fevers, no rashes, no blood tests to send people scurrying in concern. Just the slow erosion of the self, as insidious as any cancer. And, like cancer, it is essentially a solitary experience."*

When one is severely depressed, the feelings of guilt, worthlessness and helplessness are beyond belief. I blamed myself for all the problems in the world. I was always making mistakes, decisions were utterly impossible. My mantra became, "When will I ever be normal again?" and "Will I ever be normal again?" The therapist Don and I visited together assured me, *"It's just going to take time. You need to try to accept the present for what it is and try to forgive yourself."*

I couldn't believe her – this horror would never end and I knew I deserved it. Only now do I really appreciate how kind it was of Don to accompany me on those visits. He remembers them better than I do, as both depression and mania relieve a person of his memory.

I made so many mistakes. The incident with the truck was the worst. One day as we were taking equipment off the lobster boat for the winter, I thought I could please Don and back the truck down closer to the dock. My excuse when I ran it over a truly enormous granite block that wasn't even in the driveway was that the height of the truck and the car were so different that I accidentally didn't look downwards enough. Don was horrified but very kind about the accident. It must have cost a fortune, having for one thing destroyed the gas tank. How could anyone miss that block – it was huge and on the grass, not on the road. For three entire days all I could bring myself to do was apologize.

There were myriad other examples of my clumsiness and inattention. "Don," I said, "anyone could have hydroplaned the car under the back of that truck under those slick conditions. It was just an accident." "But I barely touched the back of that motorcycle on the hill – he's just making a big deal out of it to get some insurance money." My ability to hang on to things was especially alarming – coffee cups, glasses, even plates of dog food ended up on the floor, due to some sort of combination of self-consciousness, lack of concentration, or nervousness. The possibility that these problems were due to the medications did not occur to me.

Don's amazement at my behavior kept the vicious circle whirling faster and faster. We were both waiting in vain for me to be normal – it just didn't happen. My heart and my body were broken. In fact it was somewhat of a relief for me to return to the Cape – at least Don wouldn't be annoyed for a while by my countless idiocies. I knew getting away from me was good for him.

Life was as bleak as could be. Not only could I not think nor play platform tennis, I couldn't even walk right. Two friends told me, *"You're walking completely differently. Your gait has changed."* I ran into trees, tripped over easily avoided branches on paths, over obvious sills. One time, after my doctor had added a small amount of Lithium to the dosage of Depakote that I was now taking, I was on the telephone and going down the steep basement stairs. I came within an inch of careening headfirst onto the concrete. The experimental drug combination would not be tried again, but it almost killed me.

Physical frailties were confusing to my friends who went walking with me, and very embarrassing. At the little pre-school in which I was volunteering, the children naturally asked me to help them zip up their jackets – impossible. The only act I could perform for them was to tie up their shoelaces and even that sometimes had to be done twice. How they must have wondered about me, as I did, but luckily they were only five years old!

My ability to follow and participate in even simple discussions failed almost completely. No ideas filtered in, no ideas came out. What a contrast with the manic person who had had three or four brilliant ideas all stumbling over each other during a single sentence. And indeed a contrast with the reasonably intelligent person who had excelled scholastically all her life. Though I'd never had to voice my belief in my own intelligence and often wondered about it in the face of others' intellects, losing faith in holding my own in even simple chats with good friends was traumatic, to say the least.

How could anyone want to talk to someone so stupid, so boring as I was, I wondered. There was no inkling that even a small part of my brain would start working again and I was frightened. Reassurance was never enough – I knew there was nothing left of me to love. Depression is very difficult for friends, as I said – we are ultimately too needy and cannot be comforted.

In losing my verbal self I lost one of my major interests: words. Their derivations, roots, nuances, translations were prime topics at our dinner table when I was growing up (second only to politics). My fascination with Latin and the mysteries one could solve through its study and its relation to Spanish and French had continued all my life and given me much pleasure, which I often shared with Harriet. Any idea of attempting to play Boggle or Scrabble together was not even in question anymore.

Kate Millett expresses this loss so beautifully: "*During depression the world disappears. Language itself. One has nothing to say. Nothing. No small talk no anecdotes. One's real state of mind is a source of shame. So one is necessarily silent about it, leaving nothing else for subject matter. The loss of language is so crucial, such a bereavement…Yet one mourns language, sociability, camaraderie, needing it now more than ever. And how necessary it becomes just as one observes its superficiality; the wavering of friends, the coolness of strangers, the essential uncaring of life itself, its monstrosity. And in the face of this evil – not even to have words to protect one from the vacuum. To grow mute as well as helpless.*"

Processing directions was out of the question. Even the instructions given to the little pre-schoolers were incomprehensible to me. I had to fake it and rely on one six-year old who'd played the games before. Helping them do jigsaw puzzles was pretty much the best I could do, but luckily for me, they didn't really notice how debilitated I was. They loved having me around – one small piece of happiness in the dark.

Others weren't quite so understanding. Once when I asked a stranger to repeat his instructions for the fourth time, he looked at me aghast, "*Are you crazy, lady?*" Upon asking another stranger for directions, I heard him beep behind me as I turned exactly the opposite way than the one he had just indicated.

Even **written** directions were complete mysteries to

me – I could not take them in nor follow them. After five or six visits to the dentist in Boston from October to May, I was still following written directions to myself and constantly making wrong turns. (But one glorious day I realized mid-trip that the car finally seemed to know where it was going. A great cause for celebration -- no one can imagine the deep relief I felt that day. My first book title since the previous July: "May 1, 2006: The Day I Got My Brain Back.")

But for all those months, it was not a pretty sight. In public I presented a self-absorbed, morose, non-verbal stumbling figure and in private with Don my anxieties and fawning attempts to please him only increased. Upon hearing during a therapy session that he had stayed with me largely out of obligation, my shame and humiliation were complete. I sobbed uncontrollably for days. Though I deeply needed Don's reassurance that he loved me, I didn't feel it – he was still seeing himself as a *"nurse and a babysitter."* And of course in my pain I was too concerned with my self even to contemplate that he too might need to feel valued and loved.

The therapist that winter felt it was clear I knew what I needed to address, what I needed to know about Don, what to do about him. He thought it was most positive that Don was so willing to come in and to begin to process the whole experience, which he (Don) hadn't wanted to do. Though as usual I can hardly remember what we talked about, it was always interesting, often surprising. It was only during the sessions that I actually felt I had something interesting to say. A year or so later, he described me as *"likeable and articulate, though with very low self esteem."* The latter seems obvious to me, the former two adjectives really surprise me, given how I felt.

My dependence on Don and on his signs of caring for me was exaggerated but I couldn't seem to help it, even though it clearly made him uncomfortable. The small gestures of affection, the many ways a good, long marriage self-perpetuates – all gone. As he explained to the therapist, *"I've been trying hard to be nice since I know that my distance only deepens her depression, but the romance seems to have disappeared."* This strong man had had his life's assumptions thrown into question during the summer crisis and he hadn't gotten back his footing. To process with the therapist was helpful while we were actually in the office, but dealing with our shattered world and its future was going to take time.

There was nothing to do but wait. My only hope was the doctor's words that I would indeed get better. He had decided that although the Lithium had stopped the mania, it was not helping me with my depression and changed the prescription to Depakote. The change didn't make much difference -- over these months, I had become a shell, an excruciatingly boring shell.

Luckily for Don, we agreed at some point in the winter of 2006 that I could spend time alone, so he set off for two weeks by himself – some much-needed solitude in France. The pain and confusion of the last eight months had taken a terrible toll. He just wanted to think about something else for a while. The emails we exchanged while he was in his adopted country were the most honest and fruitful conversations we had had in almost a year. But we weren't out of the woods yet.

The winter continued in sadness and immobility, the depression and all its concomitant hopelessness were only exacerbated by more and more reports of my outrageous behavior and manic loss of control. An email from an acquaintance from Virginia reported he knew about the problems I'd been having, having had a talk with my friend on the Cape. Two positive strangers discussing me – how horrible. The shame, guilt and then this ultimate violation of privacy are such integral parts of the aftermath of a manic episode.

Pete Earley wrote a wonderful book, *Crazy: A Father's Search Through America's Mental Health Madness*, and quotes these words from his son: *'People don't understand how ashamed you feel because you're so different – ashamed and embarrassed and angry. I hurt people who I love when I was crazy, and now they're all scared of me.'*

Dealing with the shame and guilt when depression has taken over is virtually impossible. As I've said, whenever I could I explained and apologized, but the mountain of evidence that I was in all likelihood the worst person on earth continued to grow.

To prove something to myself, to show that I could actually make a decision, I enrolled in a language school in Mexico for two weeks – it was a disaster. Some friends had thought it might be, but no one had dared mention their concern to me, thinking that *"at least you were doing something and making a decision."* During the year as I was co-teaching an English class to a group of Brazilians,

I'd come up with so much of my old Spanish vocabulary that I felt hopeful the fluency I'd attained when working and studying in Madrid in 1968 would miraculously reappear. And during those two hours of teaching, I'd been able to throw off the overwhelming despair.

However, any hope for a moratorium on the depression while in Mexico was in vain. It was a miserable two weeks of pure loneliness, no language acuity, nothing left of the gregarious personality which normally would have drawn my fellow students into friendships. I should have declared the war over and returned early, but it would have been chickening out. It was a failure.

It was my sister Harriet, as usual, who made a big difference in lightening my mood that spring. *"I just can't understand why you won't listen to me and go to a neurologist. Your eye/hand coordination is non-existent – it's no wonder you still can't play paddle. Why are you digging in your heels on this?"* So off we went together, and immediately following a blood test the neurologist ordered to assess the level of the Lamictal I was taking, she called to report I was **way** off the charts. The amount I was taking each day was **eleven** times the amount healthy for me. As soon as I stopped the drug, my balance and coordination returned.

Even in the simplest information on the Internet and in all the studies, it is well-known that Depakote elevates the strength of Lamictal in a person's body. But the psycho-pharmacologist assured me with great equanimity that they don't test for this. I had spent all winter begging for answers to my problem with coordination and this simple fact and blood test were all that was required to restore it. He took no responsibility for it.

The shame and humiliation around my inability to play platform tennis need never have happened nor contributed to my depression. It certainly reinforces the need to question the medical information we receive from our doctors, something most of us were not brought up to do.

As late spring went into summer, the complete despair of the past many months did lift somewhat as we set out again for Maine, but it was brought back by the stress of too many guests at once. "On the one hand," I wrote late one night in the middle of the summer, "I get so lonely, on the other I cannot bear to have so many people in the house the whole time. Sometimes I have good conversations, sometimes people I'm talking with think they're having good conversations with me. I'm a great hider. If I don't hide my feelings from Don, he gets sick of it by now, not just worried." I mourned my still vain craving for hugs and signs of affection from him.

"It's the feeling of desolation, of totally not being able ever to be happy again, to be able to forget the harm I have caused, but it is still around me and I don't know if I can erase all of it in either others' minds or my own."

I've discovered in speaking with others suffering from the illness of depression that they feel the stigma of it just as strongly as those of us who are afflicted with both sides of the disease. Even seeking help from a professional, as Diane Marsh says, *"is a mark of shame."* She feels that people are punished for asking for help, which of course causes *"further humiliation of one already in pain."*

For me, the stigma is more for the manic side of the illness than the depressive. As I've said, I'm a pretty good hider. In 2007, however, I wrote that "I feel pretty confident that with the medication, I will not have another manic episode, but I don't feel so confident about warding off depression. It lasted so long, it was so incapacitating, so devastating for me. Two years of this have been indescribable."

My confidence that I would not have another episode turned out to be completely off base.

Chapter Eleven:

The Biggest Disappointment Ever

And here I truly, truly believed that after all the writing, all the research, all the interviews and acquired self-knowledge I would actually recognize the onset of mania and deal with it. No such luck, it turned out. The familiar feelings of cheer, the lessening need for sleep...it was actually all the same and **again** I didn't admit it. And now I have lost the sustaining hope that I will recognize it in the future. For three years, I was almost totally convinced – all irrevocably wrong. So much of this book was written between August of 2005 and spring of 2008 and was laced with that strong hope. What an awful, awful disease.

But I need to find some good in all this most recent disappointment – I need to re-emphasize the extreme vigilance necessary for family and friends and the imperative of the **automatic** doctor visit when even the slightest sign of an altered state of mind is noticed – before the victim gets carried away yet again and completely goes beyond judgment and control.

It happened once more in September of 2008, a few months later than usual. The signs began to appear, friends noticed oddities in emails and conversations. As usual, I grew intensely cheerful, walking up and down the driveway at dawn, coming eventually to the incredibly startling conclusion that I was finally consciously self confident – first time since the assassination of Robert Kennedy. And I knew for sure that it was his death that had caused my loss of confidence and depression. I thought I was in command of just what I was doing and thinking, but I was wrong – that I rushed back up the driveway to share the dozens of new revelations with Don was a clear sign of things spinning out of control yet again.

I was still somewhat amenable to suggestions, at least to please Don. It's questionable, though, if I would have willingly gone to see a doctor at this point, but the time had come. As Don writes, *"At this point there should have been a med doctor who saw her automatically, without having to even discuss it – as routine. I think that would have nipped it sooner and relieved us who were really concerned now. Friends here in Brooksville expressed genuine concern that all was not right. Pol was taking this 'worry' by me and our friends as something traitorous..*

A trip to Martha's Vineyard led to a few days' observation in the same hospital in Rhode Island that had turned me around in '05, but before any good could come out of it, I cleverly figured out how to spring myself. I knew it was ridiculous for me to be there. And the doctor did not judge me manic enough to take my case to court. Don drove us back to Maine, with me arguing with him unpleasantly all the way (just as in July of 2005 on the way to the wedding), and smoking like a chimney. We couldn't get along, so I went to live in the other house.

I imagine the signs were blatantly clear at this point, but I knew my friends were totally over-reacting when they encouraged blood level checks and doctors' visits – all of this as usual was infuriating since I was finally feeling so good, so brilliant and alive. One of my best and oldest friends, Betsy, arrived for a few days, calming me down somewhat and relieving Don of responsibility for a bit. But I even resented her quiet admonitions and decided to go to the Cape and see some real friends. It took all day to fill up the Prius – loaded with vegetables, clothes, paperwork, meaningful pictures, a huge plastic jar of salsa I'd made – Pascal could only have a tiny part of the back seat. Don was terrified that I was taking Pascal, but I insisted on it.

I was so tired of my sister's old cars and decided to go through Bangor to get her a new Subaru. Not so easy. Though this time I had my credit card and checkbook ready, there was some question of the insurance. While the salesman was inside trying to figure it all out and speaking with Don, I had carefully removed all the dozens of things from my car and placed them behind the new one, ready to go with Harriet's new vehicle. Who knows what I was planning to do with mine.

Pascal wandered around in great confusion, a policeman appeared and told me roughly to get everything off the tarmac post haste. Another policeman showed up and stood there silently. My plan for my sister's surprise had failed – I finally was kicked off the lot by the owner (shades of the past), Pascal was persuaded to get back in, the salesman wouldn't even shake my hand goodbye. I wonder how long it had taken them to figure out how crazy I was – probably not very.

I got into trouble again a few hours later, as I had inadvertently left my credit card at a coffee place in Bangor. As I was unable to pay for the gas I'd just poured into my car, the police were called, one of them alarmingly large and mean – finally, finally, the manager reached Don who paid with his card over the phone. The policemen seemed unconscionably rude to me – of course I knew I was behaving perfectly beautifully under the circumstances.

Two hours later, I was driving in the middle lane on Route 95 in northern Massachusetts, cruise control set at 70, when suddenly the car swerved violently to the left, then to the right and landed upside down. I thought it was very odd to be upside down, held close to the roof by the seatbelt. It was much too tight to undo. I set off the flashers, blew my horn, wondered mildly why those trucks I heard hadn't stopped to find me. I kicked out the door a bit, thought that in a while I could probably kick it further and somehow get out of the seatbelt. A voice spoke to me kindly, cut the seatbelt, pulled me bodily upwards and out. Amazingly, for the first time in eight years, I didn't think first of Pascal, who must have been terrified. She disappeared into the woods.

"So why can't I just put the Johnny on over my sweater anyway?" I demanded in the ER at the hospital in Newburyport. "My sister knitted it for me, I'm cold, and what difference does it make?" I think this is what got me in trouble – my behavior was bad enough for sedation (oh how I hated the nasty-looking woman who dealt it out -- I fought her as hard as I could). I know I wiggled out of the Velcro tying my arms to the bed, so next they used leather. End of memory.

Harriet and Don tried to give the psychiatric evaluator some of my immediate and past history and when I woke up, she apparently interrogated me carefully. Don and Harriet were amazed that the decision to keep me there was so close – it almost didn't happen.

And so ten days in another hospital, having no respect for the Latvian psychiatrist in charge of my case – another doctor making up his decisions based on nothing perceptible, forcing me to stay there far longer than need be, I thought. How I disliked him. The hospital had a few good interactive workshops, the physical setup was perfectly nice. On a day my sister Lucy came, I had decided to make up my eyes heavily to meet the doctor – she described me later to Harriet as a "monster," and "amoral." It's true – I probably did look like a monster (I don't know how to use makeup), and when manic depressives go completely out of control, amoral would be a good descriptive adjective.

Oh, it's all so discouraging – for a week or so after being released, I felt perfectly fine, glad to be alive and out of the hospital. Then, as before, the awful depression set in and continued for week after week. I spent the time desultorily making pots, playing bad paddle tennis, a picture of misery yet again, apologizing for every false move (and there were many). I tried to comfort my useless brain which again could not focus or concentrate or remember a single fact. I remembered I'd been alive, vital, super-intelligent fairly recently, so a respectable mind must lie in there somewhere. But where was it? At least this depression only lasted about two months.

Epilogue

Bi-Polar

The crap that surfaced
in the thrall
of manic strives and far flung
calls
It touched us all
and changed our lives
and soiled our norm with outlaw sides.
But underneath
and hard to see
was cutting strength
and energy
and where's the real
and who are we
that strut about
for all to see

In the end Don saw and chose the underlying strength.

We are not monsters by intention. We manic depressives are human beings with an illness that affects other people emotionally, physically, financially, usually to the detriment and/or destruction of relationships, lives, and fortunes. What I have tried to do here is to summon my own intelligence and courage to present the inside view of both sides of my illness and then the outside view of how my mania in particular intruded on the lives of so many others.

There is so much stigma attached to mental illness in general, manic depression in particular. As I have described, it is apparently unbelievably frightening to be around someone with acute mania, and without proper medication the mania only goes deeper. Though many of the causes are understood, in particular that it is a chemical imbalance in the brain, there are still differences of opinion and questions out there. At least there is much research going on and well there should be, given the millions afflicted with this disease.

It's hugely discouraging to think about the lack of any good therapy in any of the facilities in which I was incarcerated. This has to be the case for most of the other patients. My experiences with the majority of the various psychiatrists and drug dispensers make me at the very least sad and frustrated when I consider how much better my illness might have been handled and perhaps even brought to an end. My hope would be that workshops like the one on Cape Cod in 2003 might be duplicated and that kind of information be widely disseminated.

During the course of these years, I have been mostly blessed by friends who understood the illness was beyond my control. Finally recognizing, after many years of denial, that I am indeed a manic depressive and will always need to be medicated and monitored means that life has changed irrevocably. This emphatically does not mean I will stop trying to explain my illness if I come across others whom I have affected or hurt.

Close friends need to be as observant as they can. Even not so close friends need to know who has responsibility for a person with my illness and go to them with their concern – when a manic depressive, for instance, "shows up in bare feet in the snow," or acts "brassy," or "aggressively cuts a peony." A manic depressive person is not ultimately their responsibility, but they can be helpful and caring.

It usually ends up in the lap of the family. No one should be asked to do so much, and yet with this illness, families are forced into untenable situations with no way out. In my case my illness had the most impact on Don and Harriet. Those were the two who had the most responsibility for me. Harriet kept rushing to my defense, dealing with the friends I had chastised and humbled, talking to police, hospital administrators, detectives, convincing me to sign myself into hospitals. Luckily for both of us, her husband loves her and tolerated her desperate attempts to help, her constant absences and the money they spent helping me.

And Don, a last poem:

Healing

Where does the recuperation
come from
the salve for spirit, the comfort
What the hell is closure?
It only sanctifies our silly
norms of feeling –
or makes good t.v.
I wonder where I fit.
I know the balm
of Pol's return
heals to all degrees
and makes me wonder
where I've been
and how she got to me.

The harshness of this illness makes such closure indescribably difficult and many, many marriages founder. We were lucky – after a year, Don and I had come together past the mania, the depression, but nothing was easy as our hurt had been so deep. And I was so lucky that when another episode occurred in 2008, Don had already achieved his own acceptance and was ready to deal with it.

And I still don't know what my next years will be like, though I do know I will never be the same again. Manic depression will always be lurking around my own particular corner. Who could have ever guessed that such a happy little girl who spent her first 20 years just living to make people laugh could find this horror in her future. Perhaps the next 20 will be a return to that joy, a reward for making it to the other side!! Wouldn't that be wonderful. I wish it for all of us.

My real reward will be if I have succeeded in educating and informing my readers about the nature of this mean, unfair illness. If from now on you do not shudder when you see someone out of control with mania or with depression, but approach that person with understanding and compassion. That is what I want in presenting this piece. Allow a person who has confused or hurt you in his craziness to apologize and explain. Every kindness, every caring and understanding gesture will alleviate the shame and help us deal with our reality.

Bibliography

Adamec, Christina. How to Live with a Mentally Ill Person: A Handbook of Day-to-Day Strategies. New York: John Wiley and Sons, 1996

Berger, Diane, and Berger, Lisa. We Heard the Angels of Madness: One Family's Struggle with Manic Depression. New York: William Morrow, 1991

Childers, Erskine. The Riddle of the Sands. New York: Dodd, Mead and Company, 1915

Custance, John. Wisdom, Madness and Folly: The Philosophy of a Lunatic. New York: Pellegrini and Cudahy, 1952

Duke, Patty and Hochman, Gloria. A Brilliant Madness: Living with Manic-Depressive Illness. New York: Bantam Books, 1992

Earley, Pete. Crazy: A Father's Search Through America's Mental Health Madness. New York: Putnam Publishing Group, 2006

Goodwin, Frederick K. and Jamison, Kay R. Manic-Depressive Illness. New York: Oxford University Press, 1990

Hamilton, Ian. Robert Lowell: A Biography. New York: Random House, 1982

Jamison, Kay R. An Unquiet Mind. New York: A.A. Knopf, 1995

Karp, David A. Burden of Sympathy: How Families Cope with Mental Illness. New York: Oxford University Press, 2001

Kraepelin, Emil. Manic Depressive Insanity and Paranoia. New York: Arno Press, 1976

Lyden, Jacki. Daughter of the Queen of Sheba. New York: Houghton Mifflin: 1997

Manning, Martha. Undercurrents: A Therapist's Reckoning with Depression. New York: Harpercollins Publishers, 1994

Marsh, Diane T. and Dickens, Rex M. How to Cope with Mental Illness in Your Family. New York: Jeremy P. Tarcher/Putnam, 1998

Miklowitz, D.J. The Bipolar Disorder Survival Guide. New York: Guilford Press, 2002

Miklowitz, D.J. and Goldstein, M.J. Bipolar Disorder: A Family Focused Treatment Approach. New York: Guilford Press, 1997

Millett, Kate. The Loony-Bin Trip. New York: Simon and Schuster, 1990

Mondimore, Francis Mark. Bipolar Disorder: A Guide for Patients and Families. Baltimore: Johns Hopkins University Press, 1999

Solomon, Andrew. The Noonday Demon: An Atlas of Depression. New York: Scribner, 2001

Swados, Elizabeth. The Four of Us: A Family Memoir. New York: Farrar, Strauss and Giroux, 1991

Torrey, E. Fuller, MD and Knable, Michael B., DO. Surviving Manic Depression. New York: Basic Books, 2002

Wolpert, Louis. Malignant Sadness: The Anatomy of Depression. New York: Free Press, 1999

Printed in the United States
215631BV00001B/1/P

9 781440 137402